The Blood Code

Unlock the Secrets of Your Metabolism

Dr. Richard Maurer

ISBN: 0991218108
ISBN 13: 9780991218103

www.TheBloodCode.com
Beautiful Portland, Maine 04101
Tel: (800) 351-6554
E-mail: Media@TheBloodCode.com

Special discounts are available on quantity purchases by corporations, associations, and others. For details, inquire at the e-mail/number above.

Printed in the United States of America
The Blood Code™ is a trademark of Richard Maurer

Cover design by Pulp and Wire.
Content and copy edits by Genevieve Morgan and Melissa Hayes
Author photograph by Maxwell B. Maurer

At the heart of *The Blood Code* is a simple blood test panel. Test results are not to be feared; instead, they create a "GPS coordinate" that maps how your body is currently interacting with your diet and fitness habits. Once you know where you are, you can better choose the course that takes you toward disease recovery and real wellness. Here are some quotes from people, like you, after they acted upon *their* Blood Code.

After learning about my blood test results, I started doing the things that my body needed to stay healthy. As a result, I have maintained a better weight and noticed remarkable energy from the changes I made in my diet and exercise routine.
—Tony Cohutt

I recently chose to follow my Blood Code rather than take medication, and I am glad I did. My HgbA1C went from 7.4 to now-nondiabetic levels. I am lighter and healthier, and I feel great.
—Jim Gourhan

For years, I tried every thyroid prescription, thinking that if I just got the right one, I'd feel better. Finally, with no change in my prior thyroid dosage, I used the Blood Code to guide my diet and exercise. Within a few months, I was coming out of the hole I had been in for half a decade. I wish I had found Dr. Maurer's work sooner.
—Alisa Marquette

I know now that eating right—and this involves eating far more fats than I was used to—supports me in my quest for the energy I need to enjoy the challenges of the day. Today, I am back to enjoying life while making fun plans for the future, and the future is now.
—Sarah Goodwin

This approach was completely different and more on point. With the right guidance, I could easily change my food habits. Change is never easy; however, when you know it is necessary, there is no other choice. Choosing to live a longer and healthier life is a no-brainer. Thank you.
—Connie Koengeter

I saw my mother go down the road of dementia after a decade of diabetes and medications. So when my doctor said we should "watch" my blood sugars as they started to go up, I wanted to act. I saw Dr. Maurer and followed the Blood Code diet; now, my high blood sugars are gone. I feel better, and know I will live a better life in my future.
—Jeanne Tarbox

After being diagnosed with sleep apnea, and unable to lose an extra ten pounds, my blood work showed I was prediabetic. With this information I was able to target my diet and exercise and lose seventeen pounds, resolve my sleep apnea problem, and have more energy.
—Patty Hagge

I was heading toward type 2 diabetes a few years ago, until I took charge. Dr. Maurer's Blood Code is brilliant; I was able to turn it all around, and my blood sugar levels are normal again.
—Christina Hall

Contents

How to Use This Book

I have written a book that walks the line between an educational, science-based text and an accessible self-help guide. Some of you will read the book cover to cover, but most of you will jump to the sections that are important to you at the moment.

Let me explain.

After the introduction, you will get right into self-discovery work. Steps One and Two—blood test results and skin-fold caliper measurements, respectively—will help you to gather information about your current metabolism and health. You will probably reference these chapters when you have the results in front of you. Step One includes tests that have, up until now, been the domain of your intimidatingly confidential "medical chart." New terms are explained herein as simply as possible, and I've also included a glossary at the end of the book. Step Three helps you interpret what these results mean *for you*, like learning what the gauges mean on the dashboard of your car.

Steps Four, Five, and Six are the action steps that will effectively guide you toward the personalized diet, fitness, and nutritional habits that your body needs. If your fitness habits are in place, you will probably spend more time on Step Four—dietary changes. If your diet is working well, you may need to put more effort into the fitness principles from Step Five.

The "Lifestyle Habits" chapter details how the choices you make when it comes to alcohol consumption, sleep patterns, and stress management will affect your metabolism. The chapter called "Digging Deeper" is written for those who want to know more about what is going on "under the hood." I think this information is important, but not critical. (You can drive your car without knowing the details of internal combustion.)

Ultimately, this is a guidebook, but the landscape is not a fixed location—it is you. As your environment, habits, and age change, different parts of the book will be more important than others, so feel free to jump around. Further helpful resources and updates can be found at TheBloodCode.com.

Enjoy your journey toward improved and empowered health and well-being.

—Dr. Richard Maurer

Introduction: The Six Steps

Knowledge of the self is the mother of all knowledge. So it is incumbent on me to know my self, to know it completely, to know its minutiae, its characteristics, its subtleties, and its very atoms.
—Khalil Gibran

If you are like the patients I see in my office, you might be interested in reading *The Blood Code* because you have a history of heart disease in your family, and it's beginning to worry you; or, your weight is inching up, or maybe you've learned that you have high blood sugar or type 2 diabetes. Perhaps you are proactively searching for ways to optimize your energy, health, and disease prevention. Regardless, by choosing to read this book, you have taken a major step in reclaiming power over your own health, metabolism, and weight. Congratulations!

Research over the past generation has conclusively linked the prevention of chronic diseases—like cancer, cardiovascular disease, and dementia—to good dietary and exercise habits. Weight gain and blood sugar problems like type 2 diabetes are even more causally linked to your diet and fitness. Five of the top seven causes of death in the United States are from conditions inarguably related to your diet and fitness activities, so clearly, lifestyle counts. Good diet and exercise is important. But what is "good," and just what does that mean *for you?*

Authorities claim to have the answer for everyone: "Eat a low-fat diet, exercise three days a week, eat olive oil and more (but not too much) fish." The more-commercialized celebrity health-care magicians offer to cure your weight problem with a magic pill, a superfood, or a 3-minute workout. Medical advice as it pertains to your diet and fitness regimen has been excessively dumbed down to provide one blanket recommendation to the masses. Eminence-based medical advice, when the validity of a treatment relies upon the fame of the authority, has wrongly advised us on the daily decisions we make about our individual and families' food, fitness, and nutrition.

After twenty years of treating patients who have been confused, misled, and harmed by conflicting and often dead-wrong advice about how to treat a symptom, I hit a wall. I have helped patients to dramatically reduce their heart disease risk, resolve their type 2 diabetes, and recover their optimal weight and energy, all by recommending rational lifestyle changes based upon available medical tests. But patients remain perplexed as to why so many medical authorities, sometimes even their own health-care providers, push advice that clearly makes them less healthy. They ask me, "Why do I hear medical advice that contradicts what is working for me?" I have responded, in part, by writing this book, to teach and discuss a rational, self-driven program that relies on proven health metrics. My personal interest in health and metabolism helps drive my academic and professional vocation.

After my first college nutrition class thirty years ago, I pursued the answer to an ostensibly simple question: "What is a healthy diet?" In a generation of study, throughout premedical and naturopathic medical school, and two decades of practice, travel, and teaching, that question has changed. It is now "What does this individual need to stay healthy?" In other words, when faced with a new patient, I ask myself: "What diet or fitness change will help this person to move toward their perfect health and metabolism?" Headlines, popular diets, and one-size-fits-all medical wellness plans have only moved us further from this important question. How can you best assess which dietary, fitness, and nutritional habits will help you to recover your healthy weight, wellness, and longevity? The answer is not in a news headline or diet book; it is in *you*.

How your body responds to your environment, nutritional intake, and activity lies at the heart of whether you will be healthy for the long haul. Popular dietary advice for a "good diet" is rife with myths: "Low-fat is healthy," "Red meat is bad for you," and "Whole grains are much better than refined grains." Studies have proven these myths to be false, but they survive because of the *idée fixe* that surrounds them. What if you knew enough about your own body and how it responds to your daily diet and exercise that you could effectively write your own cure and wellness story?

Countless books offer one-size-fits-all diet and fitness plans, while others use questionnaires. (Where else in your life do you make major personal decisions based upon the results of a self-guided questionnaire?) You need a reliable way to understand how your body is responding to your current dietary, nutritional, and fitness habits. The changes you make need to be guided by something more accurate and meaningful than simply the fame of a program's authority figure. And here's the dirty little secret that the weight-loss and supplement industry doesn't want you to know: It's not hard to find out what your body really needs. In fact, it's really easy.

Common blood test panels combined with measurements taken by skin-fold calipers are the two simple but invaluable tools that will crack your Blood Code. You just need to learn how to use them. Like a GPS device, these test results plot where you are right now. It is your job to understand how to plan a course that will best take you from your current location to where you want to go. Future tests will reveal your progress and whether or not the changes you've made are keeping you on the right path. It's my job to be your guide.

Throughout this book, I will show you how to decipher the meaning of your own test results. It will become clear to you why there is no "magic bullet," like a miracle pill, for your metabolism. I will guide you along the way to help you find your metabolic sweet spot. Once you do, it will be yours to keep; you will have the tools to truly understand your metabolism, from the inside. The only real magic bullets I know of are your curiosity, your will, and your ability to respond to what you learn, making the necessary corrections to stay on course along the way.

The Blood Code opens the door for you to become your own health and fitness expert. I wrote it for people who are sick of the smoke-and-mirrors atmosphere of the current medical establishment. Think of this book as a big fan that is going to clear the air and let you breathe freely. So, if you want to understand yourself from the inside out, and then make the necessary changes in your diet, nutrition, and fitness habits, read on. This book is for you. If you are willing, you're now ready to unlock what you need to heal yourself and create a long-term healthy future.

The most important thing to understand is this: Your lifestyle and diet interact with your genetic code. Your health, vitality, and disease symptoms occur where these factors intersect. Your genes express a certain trait when conditions are right; whether it is good or bad is irrelevant; it is what it is. How you respond is what counts. Today's research in epigenetics and genetic expression has liberated us from the former belief that genes are a fixed entity inside us. *Epigenetics* is the study of changes in gene expression, without changing the actual DNA. You can change your genetic expression, your "disease symptoms," if you properly adjust your diet and lifestyle to be in accordance with your unique genetic traits. When your daily habits are properly matched to your genetic code, the results will be expressed in your current health and your long-term wellness. And if you have children in the future, it will also be found in their genetic expression and health.

Your first step is to get some specific common blood tests. Blood test panels are like monitors on the dashboard of a car. You can see how hard the engine is working with the tachometer; the amount of fuel in the tank, with the gas gauge; and whether your car is overheating, with the temperature gauge. Your blood test panel results indicate how your body is responding to your diet, nutrition, and fitness *right now*. To drive a car, you don't need to know the details of internal combustion, but you *do* need to know what the gauges mean. Similarly, you don't need to know the detailed interaction of your metabolism, but test results, like the gauges on the dashboard, are an easy metric that will guide you toward health recovery. The steps that follow are your driver's education classes that will help you to get the most out of the performance and longevity of your vehicle.

Conventional medical advice is too often based upon the result of one blood test—one number. When this is the case, *the number gets treated, not you.* Metabolic blood tests need to be understood as one part of a bigger picture: the result of how your genetic traits are interacting with your diet and lifestyle, right now. Together, your blood tests are a window into your metabolism—the chemical processes of your body. *Metabolism* is an abused word; weight-loss marketers usually precede it with words like *Speed up your* or *Boost your.* Your body has hundreds if not thousands of ways to adjust your metabolism depending on your health, diet, and activities on a daily basis. You can't fake out your metabolism; you need to learn how to live up to its demands. Your Blood Code will be your guide.

Countless patients over the years have come into my office with prior blood tests that indicate high triglycerides and an elevated blood sugar. Their medical advice was to "Keep an eye on it." This is similar to your auto mechanic saying, "Your brakes are ninety percent worn down and the engine is running a bit hot, but we'll just keep an eye on it for now. Call if you have a problem." Nobody wants to be stuck on the side of the highway because of a problem that could have been prevented. With neglected high blood sugars, it is not the mere dilemma of a broken-down car; it is elevated stroke risk, to name just one.

I could expand here on the innate problems of our health-care delivery system and insurance reimbursement policies in the United States; instead, I will simply conclude that true disease prevention and optimal health are not a vibrant part of the insurance and medical model. A profitable medical system relies upon the exploitation of the capital resource, and unfortunately, that's your disease—your "diagnosis"—not your health. "Medical wellness centers" have indeed sprung up within the past ten years, and arguably, that has been my practice for the past twenty years, but I think the term is more of an oxymoron. Your long-term wellness and disease prevention is really up to you, because you are the one that benefits.

Ultimately, this book is about self-discovery. Your blood tests and skin-fold caliper measurements are metrics of what is happening, not a diagnosis of what you have. For example, if you measure higher skin fold on your hip as compared to your triceps, you are storing extra calories as fat, like someone who is carbo-loading. In fact, this is a wonderfully advantageous preparation for a long endurance event in cold weather, where caloric intake is limited. It is information about what is happening; it is not a label of what you are, and should be considered a telling piece of your Blood Code, not a judgment of your character.

This may sound like semantics, but words are important. Once you understand that your weight, your cholesterol, and your blood sugars are merely the expression of how your lifestyle is interacting with your DNA—not a personality defect—you can shed a lot of blame and self-doubt. This will free you up to take back control. You are not a lazy person or glutton if you have type 2 diabetes; in fact, you have excellent energy-storage capacity that has helped your genes to survive millennia of scarcity. So give yourself a break, and get on with adapting your lifestyle to suit your survivor tendencies.

In my practice, people of many different shapes and sizes and ages and stages arrive with all kinds of conditions: migraines, restless leg syndrome, cholesterol issues, hypothyroid, weight gain, type 2 diabetes, and prediabetes. The steps in The Blood Code offer you a way to see what is happening and a plan for what to do about it. Fortunately, I have taken a dose of my own advice over the years.

Insulin and Insulin Resistance

Insulin is the primary hormone that responds to what you eat. You release insulin when you eat carbohydrates, and, to a lesser degree, protein. Insulin signals for the storage of sugars, and the making and stockpiling of fats; it helps your cells uptake proteins and magnesium. Over many generations, your body has evolved to favor the ability to build and store a little extra, by leaving some extra glucose behind, and by storing extra fats for future energy. Over 40 percent of people in the United States—more than have blue eyes—store so much extra fat and sugar that it is causing high blood pressure, high blood sugar, weight gain, and abnormal blood lipids—a constellation of symptoms that gives rise to the term *metabolic syndrome*, and leads to many chronic diseases.

In Step One, you will discover whether you are in this camp with a simple calculation of your HOMA-IR. If you already trend toward insulin resistance, you have proven you are one of the 40 percent, and without correction, you can quickly tip the scales toward fat gain and/or type 2 diabetes.

Insulin resistance, prediabetes, and type 2 diabetes are not different diseases; they are just different points on a time line. Each condition marks the same trait: a remarkable expression of generations of survival and performance.

I was a classic story of insulin reactivity as a teenager and in my early twenties. At the four-year graduate school in Portland, Oregon, National College of Natural Medicine, I was one of forty medical students in a study that compared the blood glucose effects of different types of sweeteners: rice syrup, maple syrup, honey, cane sugar, and barley malt. Following ingestion, we measured our blood sugar every fifteen minutes for two hours. (By the way, the data displayed no significant differences between the sweeteners.)

I was kept afterward because my blood glucose was below 40 mg/dL (which is very low blood sugar) at the two-hour mark. I felt okay—albeit, a bit hyper, a condition that was not unusual for me. By three hours it had recovered, slightly above 60 mg/dL, due to my body's release of stored glucose from my liver and muscles. I learned that this reactive hypoglycemia (excess drop in blood sugar) is not the opposite of type 2 diabetes; it is related. In hindsight, my vegetarian college diet, with five-grain hot cereal and vegetable juice each morning, was the wrong thing for my genetics and slightly anxious temperament.

Within the next ten years, my mother was diagnosed with type 2 diabetes, a strong family trait for her, and, of course, for me too. Identifying metabolic reactions so early in my medical career strengthened my interest in the nature of resistance and type 2 diabetes.

Throughout my thirties, I just needed to "watch my diet." I gave up boxed cereals, concentrated grains like bagels and granola, and any drinkable sugar including juice. By my early forties, I displayed a high blood sugar level, through the HgbA1C test (defined on page 37). I needed to better manage my carbohydrates, so I set carb ranges for my meals, dropping the morning jam and toast and adding spinach and butter, and eating avocados instead of pears. I also needed to practice a smarter "metabolic circuit" fitness plan that helped to further improve my insulin sensitivity. This exercise allowed my muscles to use more of the sugar/glucose that had begun to stay in my bloodstream too long. The end result today: I feel better, fitter, and healthier than at any other time in my life, and my blood sugar has dropped back into my metabolic "sweet spot." My Blood Code panel is better than it was ten years ago.

I am pretty lean; therefore, people are surprised to learn that I was "prediabetic" according to blood tests in my early forties. The truth—that over one-third of type 2 diabetics are normal to low body weight—is not a surprise to me.

I personally follow the "mild insulin resistance" guideline from Step Three (see page 82). For comparison, my mother follows the carbohydrate restriction for someone with severe insulin resistance, and she practices resistance exercises with a trainer two days per week, and walks the other days. It has been over fifteen years since she expressed type 2 diabetic numbers on blood tests. Rather than lament about what she has to do to maintain this kind of health, she says, "It's really not hard, and I feel so much better."

Insulin resistance is not a disease label. My own insulin resistance trait explains why, historically, I could "play through" without a meal and still concentrate and feel well. I can work out for one to two hours on an empty stomach and not "run out of gas." There is always enough glucose (sugar) for my brain to function. This is kind of like a supernatural power; I just need to know how to use it. People with insulin resistance, like me, are designed really well for infrequent food intake and increased physical exertion. After long bouts of exercise, it isn't carbs that I need—it's protein and fats. Dietary protein triggers enough insulin and helps me to recover and maintain my healthy and insulin-sensitive muscle mass.

At TheBloodCode.com you can view the stories of people who have used their Blood Code, some with more effort than others, to radically improve their health. The case presentations in this book and videos on the website are not some sleek before-and-after marketing pitch; they are real people who are willing to share their stories in hopes that they can help others find non-drug, self-motivated ways toward reversing diabetes, improving weight, lowering heart disease risk, and just feeling better. All the patients share a common truth: They feel more confident about their bodies and health going forward.

I recognize that it might be easier to blame suffering on something, or someone, else. Not long ago, a well-known celebrity went public with having type 2 diabetes. It struck me as odd when she said, "Diabetes is not my fault." Of course it's not your fault that you have a certain trait, no more than your eye color is "your fault." But, if your Blood Code reveals insulin resistance, and you continue to eat cereal and juice for breakfast, whose fault is that? Your blood test panel and skin-fold results do not require blind faith; they do not lie. The Blood Code allows you to discover the direction you need to take toward the health and vitality you deserve.

Ready?

The Six Steps

Step One: Get Your Blood Tests

You can get the tests done through your health-care provider or through a direct lab facility. If you use a local provider, confirm that all the required tests are included (the panels are listed in this book and on the website, TheBloodCode.com). Be sure that you will receive a copy of the actual results, not just a summary letter. The website also contains a link to our direct lab partner, SaveOnLabs. The Blood Code Discovery Panel, The Blood Code Progress Panel, and The Blood Code Thyroid Panel are remarkably affordable, and the confidential results are sent directly and securely to you. You can choose to share your results with whomever you wish once received. These results offer you a starting point of reference, or a progress check point on the map of your health journey. In the future, if we continue to take responsibility for our health and disease prevention, I expect more options will be available for affordable direct access to blood testing.

Step Two: Measure Yourself with Skin-Fold Calipers

This is optional but elegantly informative. Some trainers use skin-fold calipers; you can also buy a simple, inexpensive, yet accurate model through TheBloodCode website. Whether you are overweight or a lean athlete, skin-fold caliper measurements, done on four key parts of your body, offer an honest metric of your current fat storage, metabolic balance, and fitness. Caliper measurements can help to distinguish whether diet or fitness is currently more important for your metabolic recovery. Your weight, measured on a scale, is an inferior and inaccurate marker of your health and metabolism. It is true that pinching and measuring a skin fold intimidates some people at first, but I know the honest result will be surprisingly helpful for your health and confidence. I hope your curiosity wins out.

Step Three: Putting It All Together—IR, High Insulin, and Hypothyroid

Now it's time to self-prescribe a program that will best fit your personalized dietary and fitness needs. Your blood tests and caliper measurements provide insight into the relationship between your genetic basis, your eating habits, your fitness, and your nutrition. In this section you will unlock *your* unique Blood Code, by asking questions like: "Do I have the storage trait?" "Do I have an insulin-resistance trait?" "Do I burn calories slower than the average bear?" Your dietary and fitness needs will be spelled out based upon your blood test and skin-fold results.

Step Four: Adjust Your Blood Code Diet

It is true that most people will improve their metabolism by exchanging some dietary sugars and carbohydrates, like sweets, breads, potatoes, and fruits with leafy vegetables, traditional fats, and proteins. In Step Three, you found out how *much* you need to change—whether you require no, slight, moderate, or severe reduction in dietary carbohydrates. In this step, you will discover *why* dietary fats are a better food choice to correct insulin resistance. The Blood Code Diet helps you to personalize the carbohydrate, fat, and protein choices that are in line with what your body uniquely requires.

Step Five: Add The Blood Code Fitness Principles

Your Blood Code allows you to see whether your current activity and exercise habits are right for your healthiest and most sustainable metabolism.

It is true that the efficient and thrifty traits that were so beneficial to your ancestors do not carry the same survival value given that your lifestyle is so metabolically efficient. Even getting the mail requires a mere click of the keyboard. If you express insulin resistance or a slow thyroid function, you need to create a lifestyle that compensates for the efficiency your body is so good at. The Blood Code Fitness Principles, when put into action, help you to balance your inner metabolic tendency with your outer activity and demand.

Step Six: Ensure Your Nutritional Support

Nutritional supplements play a smaller and more supportive role in your health compared to your diet and fitness habits. After treating thousands of people over the years and working as a technical director and clinical consultant for numerous nutritional and herbal supplement companies in past decades, I have found that only a few key nutrients have withstood the test of time and research to remain invaluable parts of The Blood Code program. You might be surprised by the reasonable and non-hyped tone of Step Six; I will not kid you with fantastic claims about what a nutrient can do for you. You need to ensure that you are not deficient in key metabolic nutrients; fortunately, these deficiencies are easy to correct with a rational, research-based nutritional plan.

When you follow the steps in The Blood Code, you should feel, perform, and look better in ninety days. Whether your new dietary, nutrition, and fitness habits are working or not does not require blind faith. Measurable improvements in your blood test results and skin-fold measurements should coincide with your improved habits. Re-check The Blood Code Discovery or Progress Panel and check your skin-fold measurements. Thousands of people have done this before, whether through The Blood Code or through Dr. Maurer's office in Maine. Tell us what you think, visit the TheBloodCode.com, and join in the discussion. Thanks for choosing TheBloodCode community to be part of your self-directed and radical health discovery and recovery plan.

Step One: Get Your Blood Tests

I have been and still am a seeker, but I have ceased to question stars and books; I have begun to listen to the teaching my blood whispers to me.
—Hermann Hesse, from *Demian*

Your dietary and nutritional habits can make or break your health; you must first know about your past and present to guide you toward your healthier future. The storied Scrooge endured dreams and apparitions of the past and present to allow him to make a grand moral shift to better his own future and the future of those close to him. Your story is less grand and moral and more personal. Once you see your past and present, revealed through blood test results rather than specters, you have the potential to rewrite a part of your future, lowering the likelihood of a stroke, heart attack, Alzheimer's dementia, and many cancers. I realize that lowering the risk of a future disease is pretty abstract; fortunately, when you follow the Six Steps of The Blood Code, you will experience tangibly better energy and health in the moment.

You need to start somewhere, and Step One is a good place to begin. Essentially you need to be your own advocate: Request and get some important blood tests. Although the conventional medical establishment might find it odd and even reckless for me to give you the tools and responsibility to understand the diet and lifestyle changes that are important for you, rest assured that you are the right person for the job. Welcome to the first step.

A Panel Is Better than an Individual Test

Single blood tests rarely provide meaningful information on their own. There are very few places in science—or life, for that matter—where a single piece of data gives a meaningful and certain conclusion. "She wore glasses, so of course she was trustworthy." This example sounds absolutely absurd, but an equally irrational statement is: "He had a cholesterol of 240, so I know he was at risk for a heart attack." The single test of cholesterol loses its value when seen in the context of all the other values in your Blood Code Discovery Panel. You have permission to become your own expert, and act upon your knowledge. Step One of The Blood Code is a reference of sorts; review the parts that are important for you.

Nationally in the U.S., laboratories that perform blood tests have an obligation to get results to you, not to just the ordering practitioner. Yet, there are archaic laws in some states that restrict your access to this information about yourself, as though you can't be trusted. I can understand the concern if the blood test is a complex cancer panel that requires statistical interpretation, but a basic metabolic assessment? It's like rudimentary wiring. To pursue this example, my state law currently allows me to do basic plumbing and electrical work *in my own home* but I appropriately can't do this work in other peoples' houses for hire (I am neither a plumber nor an electrician). It follows that you can and should be trusted to view and act upon your own blood test results, but you probably should not interpret others' results for hire, unless you are a properly licensed professional.

Your doctor can be a partner in your quest to get these tests done and results in your hands. And at TheBloodCode.com, you can find a link to the most accessible and affordable direct laboratory facility within the U.S. I anticipate greater direct consumer access to self-ordered blood testing over the next several years, especially with the new technology of performing blood tests on ever-smaller samples.

Practical science relies on the famous Einstein adage, *"Make things as simple as possible, but not simpler."* I know there will be medical colleagues who will think The Blood Code Panels are too much information for the average person, while others will claim that some specialized tests have been left out. The following Panels provide you with the maximum information about your health and metabolism while maintaining an affordable and understandable interpretation. Anything less would be "simpler."

These tests are not proprietary. They are of equal quality at any legitimate laboratory facility. If you do the panel through your health-care provider, be sure that all tests are included—and get the results rather than a summary letter. The following test panels have been honed to include the essential tests that provide you with meaningful, actionable information.

Throughout this book, reference ranges will first list U.S. standard units, as of the end of 2013—then International S.I. units will be listed in parentheses. Lab results from clinical cases are reported in U.S. standard units. A conversion chart can be found on page 53, and is available at TheBloodCode.com.

Ready? Let's get on with your results.

The Blood Code Discovery Panel

Everyone should start with The Blood Code Discovery Panel, which includes all of the tests necessary to assess which direction your metabolism is going, such as excess storage, insulin resistance, and subsequent inflammation. The Discovery Panel includes your vitamin D and ferritin. The reasons will be explained under each individual test. The

Blood Code Discovery Panel helps you to thoroughly evaluate how your current diet, fitness, and nutrition interact with your genetic traits and environment. The Discovery Panel is your first step.

Preparation: Fast for 10 to 16 hours, overnight. Drink enough water, and take your prescribed medications.

1. Complete Blood Count with Differential [CBCD]
2. Comprehensive Metabolic Panel
3. HgbA1C
4. Serum Insulin
5. Lipid Panel
6. 25 OH Vitamin D
7. Ferritin

The Blood Code Progress Panel

The Blood Code Progress Panel is an affordable follow-up panel that you can do on a quarterly basis each year to ensure that your progress is in-line with your true health potential. The diet, fitness, and nutritional steps that you implement should provide you with measurable improvements. If your vitamin D and ferritin were okay on your Discovery Panel, the Progress Panel is all you'll need going forward. The Progress Panel is an objective beacon that ensures you are on the road toward a longer and healthier life.

Preparation: Fast for 10 to 16 hours, overnight. Drink enough water and take your prescribed medications.

1. Complete Blood Count with Differential [CBCD]
2. Comprehensive Metabolic Panel
3. HgbA1C
4. Serum Insulin
5. Lipid Panel

Definitions of the Tests in The Blood Code Discovery and Progress Panels

1. **Complete Blood Count (aka, CBC or Hemogram) with Differential:** To ensure a normal and healthy blood count. Anemia can alter HgbA1C results.
2. **Comprehensive Metabolic Panel (CMP):** Contains several markers, most importantly:
   - Liver enzymes—May show benign fatty liver disease, a condition where high insulin causes sugar to get stored as fat in the liver.
   - Fasting glucose—Also referred to as *blood sugar,* this is your pre-food baseline of circulating blood glucose prior to eating.
3. **HgbA1C / HbA1c (Hemoglobin A1C):** Also known as *glycosylated hemoglobin,* this subset of the hemoglobin molecule is part of a calculation that reflects your eight- to twelve-week average blood glucose. A useful tool to assess the changes in your blood sugar from changes in dietary and exercise habits over a period of months.
4. **Serum Insulin:** Your sensitivity or resistance to this anabolic hormone tells an important story about your disease risk. Your fasting glucose and fasting insulin together create a calculation called HOMA-IR. The important part is the "IR," which stands for *insulin resistance.* Your HOMA-IR calculation is an invaluable tool used to help identify your need and response to dietary and exercise habits, and their impact on your health.
5. **Lipid Panel:** Provides the Triglyceride:HDL-cholesterol (TG:HDL) ratio, a strong indicator of heart disease risk.
6. **25 OH Vitamin D:** While cause and effect is still up in the air, insulin resistance is strongly associated with low vitamin D status.

7. **Ferritin:** This is the storage form of iron; too low, and you have significant iron deficiency. But while it is necessary for muscle function and manufacture of blood cells, high levels indicate inflammation or a genetic iron storage condition.

The Blood Code Thyroid Discovery Panel

Thyroid hormones are part of what regulates your metabolic rate, especially when you are not physically active. It is understandable why doctors suspect the thyroid gland may be responsible when you have a "sluggish metabolism." Far from acting on its own, your thyroid gland responds to dietary and environmental conditions, and if you are prone to insulin resistance, hypothyroid can be in the mix as well.

Insulin resistance and hypothyroid are intimately connected. Recent research has determined that insulin resistance raises the incidence of thyroid problems.[1][2] As I have said already, historical lifestyle is a major player; if your ancestors burned the metabolic candle at both ends by combining a lot of physical demand with low caloric intake, they created the perfect environment for these two conditions to develop together, and you are the brilliant representation of that survival.

Not everyone needs his or her thyroid thoroughly tested. If you have no family or past history of thyroid problems, past screening tests have been normal, the Thyroid Discovery Panel is not necessary for you.

If a thyroid problem is suspect, due to your family history or past abnormal test, answers are better than hunches. The all too common symptoms of hypothyroid include fatigue, weight gain, constipation, coldness, and dry skin. The Blood Code Thyroid Discovery Panel provides information that is beyond typical thyroid screening. It offers you and your health-care provider a better sense of whether the thyroid is part of your metabolic imbalance.

Preparation: The thyroid panel does not require fasting, *but exercise can significantly alter levels of circulating thyroid hormones.* A morning, pre-exercise, fasting blood draw is convenient. Drink enough water, and take all medication as prescribed by your health-care practitioner.

1. TSH (Thyroid Stimulating Hormone)
2. Free T4 (Free Thyroxine)
3. Free T3 (Free Triiodothyronine)
4. TPO antibody (Thyroid Peroxidase)

Definitions of the Tests in The Blood Code Thyroid Discovery Panel

1. **Thyroid Stimulating Hormone (TSH):** This hormone comes from higher in your brain (the pituitary gland). TSH quantifies whether the pituitary is whispering or yelling at the thyroid to produce adequate T4 and T3. If it is yelling (i.e., your number is higher), it is a sign that the thyroid gland is producing inadequate hormone.
2. **Free Thyroxine (Free T4):** The primary hormone that your thyroid produces, T4 is actually a pre-hormone, since the activity only occurs when it is converted into T3 inside your cells.
3. **Free Triiodothyronine (Free T3):** The activated form of the thyroid hormone that helps to regulate the BMR in all your cells. Numerous enzymes adjust and control the amount of conversion from T4 to active T3 and the final deactivation of T3.
4. **Thyroid Peroxidase (TPO antibody):** This test quantifies the amount of antibody—a protein of your immune system—that can "knock out" some of your thyroid gland's activity, usually causing it to produce less thyroid hormone over time. If people have hypothyroid findings *and* elevations in this antibody, prescription treatment will likely begin sooner rather than later.

You will notice that there is no *Progress Panel* for thyroid. If there are abnormalities in the Thyroid Discovery Panel, you will want to develop a strategy for follow-up testing with your health-care provider. Follow-up thyroid tests are best done a la carte. I have clients for whom I only order TSH to assess progress; others need the TSH with free T4 and/or free T3. In my opinion, the TPO antibodies rarely need to be retested once they are checked once.

Evaluate Your Discovery and Progress Panel Results

All meanings, we know, depend on the key of interpretation.
—George Eliot (pen name of savvy English author, Mary Anne Evans)

This is as good a time as any to reiterate: This book is not intended to be a substitute for medical advice and intelligent diagnostics. There are other disease considerations that arise given abnormal blood test results. The information given here is designed to help you to better understand yourself and to make informed decisions about your diet, fitness, and nutritional habits. Insight you gain about yourself and improvements in your health should strengthen, not replace, the relationship you have with your health-care provider(s).

1. Complete Blood Count with Differential (CBC, Hemogram)

The CBC has several different components related to your white blood cells (WBC) and red blood cells (RBC). The RBC values will check for the presence of anemia, which mimics so many metabolic conditions, like hypothyroid, and can complicate the blood tests used for blood sugar control.

White blood cells (WBC or leukocytes)
3–10 M/uL is normal (S.I. units are the same)

White blood cells are the collective of cells that form your immune response to infection and participate in inflammation and allergy reactions. The lower the number, the less total white blood cells cruising through your bloodstream at the time of the blood draw.

Low WBC: If you were not sick at the time, the number should be on the low side of normal. Slightly lower than 3 is normal for some, but less than 2.5 should be discussed with your health-care provider.

High WBC: If the number is on the high side of normal, your immune system is probably mobilized and active, doing what it should do—fighting an infection before it even gets a stronghold in your body. If it is above 10, you were either fighting an infection or had been exposed to something. The differential contains the "count" of WBCs, and gives an indication of whether they are mostly the cells that fight viruses (lymphocytes) or the kinds of cells that mostly fight bacteria (neutrophils). The eosinophil is usually elevated if you have allergies, primarily airborne-type allergies.

Studies have linked chronically high WBCs with inflammation and heart disease risk. In population studies, people with higher body fat and poor fitness habits are more likely to have higher WBC counts and associated heart disease. If this was an issue for you, despite that WBC levels vary a little from test to test, your value should improve and lower as you gain fitness condition and lose body fat. Again, a high WBC can also indicate other non-metabolic conditions, so abnormalities should be discussed with your health-care provider.

Red blood cells (RBC or erythrocytes)
4–6 M/uL is normal (S.I. units are the same)

Red blood cells make up 40 to 50 percent of your total blood volume, moving oxygen in and carbon dioxide out of your cells. There is an iron molecule at the center of each RBC. This test is a "count" of your red blood cells. Average is 5 million cells per uL volume. Men are usually higher (4.0–5.8) and women are usually lower (3.8–5.4). Athletes want to be on the higher sides of normal, since these cells fuel your aerobic activity.

Low RBC: This signifies anemia—too few red blood cells. Your ferritin test, the storage form of iron in your body, will show whether this is the cause.

High RBC: This is not common, and might be within normal limits for you. Ferritin should be checked to ensure it's not too high.

Hematocrit (HCT)
Normal Range:
For women: 35–47% (0.35–0.47)
For men: 40–52% (0.4–0.52)

HCT is the percentage of whole blood that is red blood cells. The nickname "Crit" has become infamous, as athletes illegally and unhealthily dope with drugs that stimulate bone marrow production of RBCs, thereby giving them a higher percentage of oxygen-carrying red blood cells.

Low and high levels offer the same screening as the RBC.

Hemoglobin (HGB)
Normal Range:
For women: 11–15 g/dL (110–150 g/L)
For men: 13–17 g/dL (130–170 g/L)

HGB is the inside part of a RBC. It is made from the mineral iron and is B12-dependent. If deficient, it can affect the accuracy of interpreting HgbA1C levels.[3][4]

Low Hgb: Anemia with low HGB is usually iron deficiency, and could also be low vitamin B12. The ferritin level will confirm iron status.

High Hgb: This is rarely problematic, and should be addressed like high RBC.

Mean corpuscular volume (MCV)
80–100 fL is normal (S.I. units are the same)

MCV is a measurement of the average size of your red blood cells.

Low MCV: This signifies small red blood cells, and usually means iron deficiency.

High MCV: This results commonly from B12 deficiency. Some people have numbers that normally remain outside the reference ranges; in this case, the value remains unchanged despite nutritional improvement.

Mean corpuscular hemoglobin (MCH) and mean corpuscular hemoglobin content (MCHC): These calculations give the mathematical average HGB per red blood cell. Both tests help to tease out the different types of anemia. These tests are not metabolically pertinent, and if abnormal, should be further evaluated by your health-care provider.

Platelets (PLT)
140–400 x1000 uL is normal (S.I. units are the same)

Platelets are the cells that allow for normal clot formation. Like MCH, this test is not relevant to your metabolism, but if the number is out of the reference range, it could indicate one of many serious conditions. This should be discussed with your health-care provider.

Summary of your CBC: Ensure that you are not anemic. Even mild anemia prevents normal exercise recovery, and causes symptoms that mimic a "sluggish metabolism." Anemia is a common symptom for many non-metabolic diseases, so be sure that the results of your tests are part of an intelligent dialogue with your health-care provider.

---

2. Comprehensive Metabolic Panel (CMP)

The CMP contains screening tests for many different organ systems. For your Blood Code you will observe the ones listed below.

Fasting glucose (blood sugar)
75–95 mg/dL is optimal (4.2–5.3 mmol/L)
<75 mg/dL is too low (<4.2 mmol/L)
96–100 mg/dL is borderline (5.3–5.6 mmol/L)
101–125 mg/dL is high blood sugar, but not "yet" diabetic (5.7–7.0 mmol/L)
>125 mg/dL is diagnostic of diabetes (>7.0 mmol/L)

> **Low blood glucose,** also known as *hypoglycemia,* means that your body can't liberate the stored sugars very effectively. This was a fasting test, so it is not vulnerable to your most recent meal. Weight loss, very low-fat diets, and some drugs can result in low blood sugar. When hypoglycemic, your body will tend to break down more proteins, a state of catabolism.[5]

> **High blood glucose,** also known as *hyperglycemia,* implies that you have some insulin resistance. The degree of insulin resistance is directly associated with how high the fasting blood sugar is over 100 mg/dL (>5.6 mmol/L). A fasting blood sugar >125 mg/dL (>7mmol/L) is diagnostic of type 2 diabetes, but the earlier you can catch the elevated blood sugar *before* it is type 2 diabetes, the better. Insulin resistance, even at the early stages, is associated with serious disease risks.[6]
> Your body has this wonderful ability to release extra blood sugar in the first morning hours. Some people have a slightly high fasting blood glucose in the morning, but will discover a normal HgbA1C (blood sugar average over time); this can be explained by the "dawn

phenomenon," which is caused by the release of adrenaline and met-abolically stimulating compounds upon rising.

Non-Insulin-Resistant Reasons for High Fasting Blood Sugar:
- If you don't get "enough" sleep, you will have an extra high dawn phenomenon due to the increase of adrenaline when you get insufficient sleep.
- If you tend toward anxiety or panic, you might release excess adrenaline and therefore have an extra high dawn phenomenon.
- If you had a strenuous workout before the blood draw, your body will have released extra blood sugar from your muscles.

Liver Enzymes AST and ALT
AST and ALT 0–40 U/L is normal (S.I. units are the same)

Some labs still use the very old names ALT = SGPT and AST = SGOT. These enzymes indicate the rate of turnover of liver cells.

High liver enzymes imply that there is inflammation or irritation in your liver. The AST is more vulnerable to short-term influences, like alcohol intake or medications such as ibuprofen and acetaminophen taken within a few days prior to the test. Whereas the ALT indicates the long-term processes over weeks or months, like when your liver gets bogged down with too much fat storage, aka, fatty liver disease, or the more medical-sounding benign hepatic steatosis.

Many medications cause harmful liver irritation. If you show an elevation in your liver enzymes, and are on a prescribed or over-the-counter medication, discuss the results with your prescribing practitioner.

Creatinine and Blood Urea Nitrogen (BUN)

Normal Ranges:

Creatinine: 0.5–1.3 mg/dL (44–115 umol/dL)

BUN for women: 6-21 mg/dL (2.1–7.5 mmol/L)

BUN for men: 8–24 mg/dL (2.8–8.6 mmol/L)

Creatinine is a by-product of your muscle metabolism and is produced at a fairly constant rate; it is also eliminated at a comparable rate through the kidneys. If you have a more-advanced case of insulin resistance or history of high blood pressure, your practitioner may look at your creatinine and BUN levels to assess the kidney function. Generally, if creatinine is above normal, your kidney function should be evaluated further with a more-accurate test administered by a medical specialist. The most damaging compound to the kidney is excess sugar, so control of insulin resistance is critical when kidney function is compromised.

BUN is another compound that is a normal part of protein breakdown and protein digestion, and is regularly excreted through the kidney.

Low BUN is usually found in two very different populations: children, who have low BUN in part because of their relatively efficient kidney function; and malnourished adults, such as those on very low-protein diets.

High BUN may be due to dehydration first thing in the morning, so use this test as a reminder to stay hydrated. A protein-rich diet can also result in a slightly higher BUN level. Very high protein diets and people who use protein powders may have a BUN above 30 mg/dL (>10.7 mmol/L); this is not healthy, and dietary patterns should change.

There are other components of the CMP test panel that are not an integral part of your Blood Code. If overt abnormalities exist, discuss them with your health-care provider.

3. Hemoglobin A1C (Hgb A1C)

4.5–5.7% is normal (26–39 mmol/mol)
< 5.6% is optimal (< 38 mmol/mol)
5.8–6.4% indicates significant insulin resistance (40–46 mmol/mol)
>6.4% indicates diabetes (>46 mmol/mol)

Hemoglobin A1C (HgbA1C) is a calculation that measures a chemical reaction to hemoglobin (Hgb) in your bloodstream. Significant abnormalities in your Hgb levels, such as anemia, can disrupt the accuracy of the HgbA1C test. Fasting blood glucose measures your blood sugar only at the moment of the draw; HgbA1C measures the prior eight- to ten-week average blood sugar. In 1990, most labs reported anything below 6.5% as normal. Now, the top edge of acceptable normal is 5.7% (39 mmol/mol). This lower acceptable limit is due to mounting evidence over the years that *non-diabetic* individuals with HgbA1C between 5.5% and 6% (37–42 mmol/mol) had significantly greater stroke and cardiovascular disease than those who maintained numbers between 5% and 5.5% (31–37 mmol/mol). Furthermore, as HgbA1C numbers went above 6% (42 mmol/mol), heart disease risk correspondingly increased with each level of elevated average glucose.[7]

Low HgbA1C is very rare; I have seen it twice in clinical practice. It indicates frequent hypoglycemia and subsequent tendency toward loss of muscle tone.

High HgbA1C is directly related to blood sugar; the higher the value, the higher your average blood sugar, and subsequently, the higher your chronic disease risk. This is a very useful test to see the improvement and progress with diet and fitness changes over an eight- to ten-week period of time.

4. Serum Insulin

Fasting Insulin for adults: The ranges listed here are quite different than the wide range the lab provides on your report. The international S.I. unit conversion is based on the most scientifically validated conversion value to date: 1 uIU/mL = 6 pmol/L.[8]

Low is <3 uIU/mL (<18 pmol/L)
Optimal 3–8 uIU/mL (18–48 pmol/L)
High is >8 uIU/mL (>48 pmol/L)

First, look at your absolute insulin level; low, normal, or high. Then you can run the calculation HOMA-IR (see below) to discover the extent of your insulin resistance (chronic disease risk) or insulin sensitivity (vital and healthy metabolism).

> **Low insulin:** Labs cannot currently detect insulin lower than 2 uIU/mL. The result is reported as "below detectable limits." If there is no detectable fasting insulin, <2 uIU/mL (<12 pmol/L), and the blood sugar is significantly elevated, such as with a HgbA1C >6.2% (>44 mmol/L), this could be type 1 diabetes, and should be immediately reviewed by a doctor. There is an adult-onset type 1 diabetes called LADA, sometimes referred to as diabetes type 1.5; more-advanced blood tests, including antibody tests, can help to evaluate for the presence of this condition, and should be done through your health-care provider.

With low insulin, you can readily break down fats that you have stored. In my practice, I see low insulin with:

- people with inadequate absorption of calories;
- people who over-exercise/over-train without adequate time off to recover; and
- people who have chosen a very low-carbohydrate diet, despite having no evident insulin resistance.

High insulin: High insulin on a fasting blood test means you are in an anabolic state—effectively building fat and muscle. High fasting insulin is rare in a thin and frail person. Future risk of type 2 diabetes begins to go up in those with fasting insulin above 8 uIU/mL

(48 pmol/L). Uncorrected high insulin will usually, over time, result in insulin resistance; therefore, you need to assess your HOMA-IR for any insulin resistance.

Insulin levels during childhood and pregnancy: It is normal for growing children and pregnant women to have a slightly higher insulin level, up to 15uIU/mL (90 pmol/L). Gestational diabetes is not a condition that happens "out of the blue"; instead, it is the appropriate pregnancy-related elevation of insulin that puts some women over the top of their previously hidden insulin resistance.

HOMA-IR, The Insulin Resistance Calculation: Insulin x Glucose ÷ 405

The HOMA-IR calculation requires U.S. standard units. To convert from international S.I. units:
Insulin: pmol/L to uIU/mL, divide by (÷) 6
Glucose: mmol/L to mg/dL, multiply by (x) 18

Optimal Range: 1.0 (0.5–1.4)
Less than 1.0 means you are insulin-sensitive which is optimal.
Above 1.9 indicates early insulin resistance.
Above 2.9 indicates significant insulin resistance.

HOMA-IR = Insulin x Glucose ÷ 405
For example:
fasting insulin = 10 uIU/mL
fasting glucose = 100 mg/dL
10 x 100 = 1000, divided by 405 = about 2.5 = early insulin resistance

HOMA-IR stands for Homeostatic Model Assessment of Insulin Resistance. The meaningful part of the acronym is the "insulin resistance" part. This calculation marks for both the presence and extent of any insulin resistance that you might currently express. You can visit

TheBloodCode.com to plug in your values and get the calculation. It is a terrific way to reveal the dynamic between your baseline (fasting) blood sugar and the responsive hormone insulin.

Low HOMA-IR means that you are sensitive to insulin. A small amount of the hormone insulin is doing the trick to keep your blood sugars in good balance.

High HOMA-IR relates to your level of insulin resistance. The higher the number, the more resistant you are to the message of insulin. If you are above 2, your self-prescribed diet and fitness habits will bring your number down into the lower insulin-sensitive range. The upcoming steps direct you toward the changes that are right for you.[10]

5. Triglyceride (TG) and High-Density Lipoprotein (HDL) from the Lipid Panel

As individual tests:
Triglyceride (TG): Optimal is 40–100 mg/dL (0.45–1.1 mmol/L)
HDL: Optimal is men>44 mg/dL (>1.14 mmol/L), women>50 mg/dL (>1.3 mmol/L)

TG is the fat that is in circulation in your bloodstream; this represents a lot of caloric availability. Remember, this was a fasting test, so this does not represent your last meal. Instead, fasting TG displays the capacity for your body to make and store fats, usually at the insistence of the hormone insulin.

Low TG, <40 mg/dL (<0.45 mmol/L), shows that you are running lean; while this is good to an extent, it leaves little room for error. If times get tough, like a strenuous workout that lasts over an hour, you will start to break down. Like someone with a level of insulin that's too low, you may have trouble adding muscle mass and strength.

Post-workout meals are vital when in this category. A vegetarian exerciser with low TG is on a dangerous road toward tissue and immune breakdown (catabolism).

High TG, >100 mg/dL (>1.1 mmol/L), implies that you have done a fabulous job storing up for the big event . . . that never happened. No doubt you have plenty of fat stored in your liver, too, but the TG measured was merely the overflow. High insulin is usually behind the steering wheel of your metabolism when you have high TG. The upcoming steps will swiftly correct this excessive fat storage.

HDL on its own: The HDL represents how well your liver is producing the useful and healthful HDL-cholesterol. If you have high TG, your HDL is probably lower than it should be for your optimal health. Conversely, as you move toward a healthier metabolism, your TG will reduce and your HDL will go up. The ratio between the two is important.

TG:HDL Ratio: A More-Accurate Heart Disease Risk Assessment

This ratio, like HOMA-IR, requires U.S. standard measurements; therefore you must convert into U.S. standard units.
- *HDL: mmol/L to mg/dL: multiply by (x) 39*
- *TG: mmol/L to mg/dL: multiply by (x) 89*

Optimal range: 0.5–1.9
Some insulin resistance: 2.0–3.0
Significant insulin resistance and heart disease risk is found at ratios >3.0

TG:HDL ratio is calculated on a fasting lipid profile. Simply take the Triglyceride and divide by the HDL; the closer to one, the better.

For example: TG = 120 mg/dL and HDL=40 mg/dL. 120 / 40 = 3.0, and indicates an elevated risk of heart attack and stroke.

Low TG:HDL is desirable. As long as the TG is not below 40, your ratio can be below 1:1, as it is in many well-trained and properly nourished athletes, for example a TG of 50 mg/dL and HDL of 80 mg/dL provides a low TG:HDL ratio of 0.6.

High TG:HDL, especially >3, indicates significant risk of heart attack and stroke. I realize that high cholesterol, especially LDL, gets most of the press, and I am realistic in blaming the pharmaceutical industry for promoting this hype. The research and relevance about the TG:HDL ratio is detailed further in the "Digging Deeper" chapter.

6. Total Vitamin D (25-OH vitamin D) (Part of the Discovery Panel)

30–60 ng/mL is your optimal range. (75–150 nmol/L)

Vitamin D level in your blood can be associated with insulin resistance. There is both a synergistic effect and some cause and effect noted in the literature related to obesity, insulin resistance, and low serum vitamin D. If you show any level of insulin resistance, you want to ensure that your vitamin D is within optimal range. Some additional supplemental vitamin D can be a very important part of your metabolic recovery.

Low vitamin D: This is associated with insulin resistance, and some cause and effect is noted in the research. Therefore, if you are over-weight *and* have low vitamin D, your prognosis is worse. The take-home message: Guarantee that you are not vitamin D–deficient when you begin your journey toward a healthier weight and metabolism.[11]

High vitamin D: Too much of a good thing is too much. In clinical prac-tice, the only times I saw vitamin D levels above 70 ng/mL (>175 nmol/L) were in people who supplement with a high-dose nutritional supplement. Vitamin D has received a lot of hype in the past decade. Research has repeatedly linked low blood levels of vitamin D with many diseases. Nutritional advice by many experts fell victim to the common error in science, which is to see the tree and not the forest, or, in other words, to mistakenly see direct cause and effect where there is only an association. Low vitamin D can cause problems, clearly, but once the basic deficiency is resolved, high vitamin D can cause similar problems, like calcification and hardening of arteries. If your vitamin D is above the reference range, look for where you might be inadvertently getting excess, such as dairy products and other combination nutritionals. A good, all-around daily supplemental dosage is between 600 and 1200 IU, and should be taken in an oil-soluble form, such as with fish oil. Over 2000 IU per day should only be pursued with proper medical advice.[12]

7. Ferritin (Part of the Discovery Panel)

Normal Ranges (S.I. units are equal numbers as ug/L):
For women: 30–150 ng/mL
For men: 50–300 ng/mL
Athletes, both men and women: Raise the lower level of your normal ranges by 20 ng/mL

Ferritin is an iron-containing protein and is the primary form of storage iron in your body. The iron molecule represents your iron reserves. Animals, including humans, concentrate iron in their blood cells. When iron is in short supply, the body will rob ferritin from muscles and bones to feed the production of blood.

Low ferritin occurs when the iron reserves have been drained and not replenished. Anemia does not occur until the late stages of low ferritin, so you can still have a low ferritin even if your RBC is normal. When low, your muscles do not recover well from exertion, and you will start to experience fatigue, lack of stamina, and restless leg syndrome with insomnia. These conditions are remarkably easy to cure with iron-rich nourishment. Women are more vulnerable to this condition due to the loss of iron with decades of menstrual cycles. If you are under the age of thirty, you should add a supplemental chelated iron while looking for ways to get some iron-rich foods back into your diet (e.g., red/dark meats, bone broths, oysters, and liver).[13]

High ferritin is known to be associated with obesity and especially fatty liver with high triglycerides. Individuals with higher serum ferritin levels are more likely to have severe insulin resistance, and vice versa.[14]

"Genetic" high ferritin: Everyone should have a ferritin run at least once in his or her early to mid-adult life. A condition called hereditary hemochromatosis presents in about 2 to 4 percent of the population in the United States. This set of gene mutations triggers excess storage of iron, a trait that could have been a survival boon historically for women to survive blood loss from childbirth, but excess iron can cause a chronic inflammation and liver damage in men and postmenopausal women.

If you have levels of ferritin above 300, you need to rule out whether this is secondary to inflammation, liver problems, or hereditary hemochromatosis. Follow-up genetic tests and discussion with your health-care provider are important steps you must take to evaluate a more serious, inflammatory reason for the elevated ferritin. If ferritin is high due to insulin resistance and fatty liver, the number will improve as you implement the dietary and fitness changes from the coming steps.

The common "inflammation" test, called hs-CRP, is an optional test you can order or discuss with your health-care provider. Below I explain why this test is optional.

Optional Test: C-Reactive Protein (CRP or hs-CRP)

Optimal Range <1 mg/L

CRP is one of the proteins responsible for inflammatory processes, such as the cleanup of dead cells and bacteria. Thus, when you are sick with an infection, CRP levels appropriately go up quickly. Then, several days following infection, they should go back to very low, or below detectable, limits. It is when people carry around high baseline levels of CRP that heart disease risk goes up.

> **High CRP** is associated with an increased risk of heart disease and stroke in those with baseline CRP levels above 2.4 mg/L compared to people who were below 1 mg/L.[15]

Compounds from fat cells regulate CRP production in the body; this may be why insulin resistance and weight gain tend to associate with high CRP. Thus, CRP does not raise the risk of developing diabetes; it's simply that the underlying insulin resistance triggers the elevated CRP.[16] Baseline CRP >2 mg/L is just one more sign that you are on the road to insulin resistance and excessive fat storage. There are drugs and herbs that lower CRP, but if you lower CRP and do not correct your insulin resistance, you will have gained nothing.

Therefore, hs-CRP is really a "tagalong," $30 to $35, lesser, ancillary test. An elevated CRP piggybacks insulin resistance. CRP is often done in other medical settings, so it is worth discussing here, but the other markers within The Blood Code Panels are superior at steering your self-discovery.

> The Blood Code Test Panels are designed to be the most effective and cost-efficient way to evaluate your metabolic health and progress. Consider the Discovery and Progress Panel contents as the minimum to be done to provide useful insight; *extra* tests can be ordered at the discretion of you and your health-care provider.

Evaluate Your Thyroid Panel Results

Again, this test panel is optional, and should be run only if you or your health-care provider suspects a current or past thyroid problem.

Your thyroid gland sits just below your Adam's apple and releases some of the hormones that manage your basal metabolic rate (BMR). This is the rate of cellular biological processes at your baseline, which means without any exercise or effort, or "at rest." The simple term used to describe an underactive thyroid gland is *hypothyroid;* this condition makes up over 80 percent of people "treating" a thyroid condition. If for some reason your thyroid gland produces excessive thyroid hormone, the condition is called *hyperthyroidism.* If you have a family history of thyroid problems, a direct family member who has or had hyper- or hypothyroidism, there is greater likelihood that this gland is affecting your metabolic recovery—you therefore should be appropriately evaluated. Hyperthyroidism is a medically complicated condition and needs to be evaluated with your health-care provider. Throughout *The Blood Code,* you will learn how to better understand and manage the symptoms of a slow/hypo/sluggish thyroid.

1. Thyroid-Stimulating Hormone (TSH)

Optimal Range 0.4–4.0 uIU/mL
S.I. units are equal numbers stated as mIU/mL

TSH is the hormone from the pituitary gland in the brain that tells your thyroid gland to produce more or less of the pre-hormone, T4, and active T3. The over-simplified mechanism goes like this: Elevated TSH occurs when the pituitary gland yells louder to get the thyroid gland to produce more hormone, like a parent speaking louder to an unresponsive child to get the desired response. Conversely, if TSH levels are normal or low, the pituitary gland perceives plenty of thyroid activity in the body, and therefore has no need to use a loud voice. TSH is the most frequently used hormonal test in any conventional medical setting and is the common test to screen for thyroid function.

But TSH is controversial. Over the past twenty years, higher TSH has been linked to heart disease risk. People with slightly elevated TSH, *even within normal range,* appear to have more heart disease and higher weight than those in the lower range of normal. This has led to a dangerous trend toward overprescribing thyroid hormone to lower TSH. TSH elevation is *associated* with heart disease risk, but does not cause it. Researchers, within the past five years, have attributed the heart disease risk and weight problems of slightly high TSH to <u>insulin resistance</u>—not a thyroid condition at all.[17] TSH levels vary up and down one unit as a result of short-term exercise, so subtle changes within normal range are expected.[18] Furthermore, slightly high TSH, 3 to 6 uIU/mL, appears to be associated with longevity in those over the age of sixty-five.[19] [20] A rational evaluation of the thyroid panel, starting with TSH, follows here.

Your TSH ranges

<.02–0.4 uIU/mL: Talk to your health-care provider if your numbers are in this low range. This indicates an overactive thyroid, and occurs when your thyroid gland, or a part of your thyroid gland, starts producing too much thyroid hormone. It also occurs if you are taking too much prescription thyroid hormone.

0.4–4.0 uIU/mL: This is the "normal range." TSH fluctuates up or down 1.0 unit throughout the day; thus, the range is more important than to expect an exact number. The upper range of normal, 3 to 4 uIU/mL, can signify insulin resistance, and this number will come downward if you correct your metabolism with your prescribed dietary and fitness habits.[21] Even short-term exercise can raise TSH levels, thus the need to avoid significant exercise in the hours prior to your blood draw.

4.0–6.0 uIU/mL: This elevated TSH *might* indicate mild hypothyroid, but could also be elevated due to the combined effect of insulin resistance. TSH levels can enter this borderline range in women near menopause. This is due to the combination of several effects. During menopause, the pituitary gland releases extra LH and FSH hormones, and as the adage goes, a rising tide lifts all ships—the TSH elevates as well. Furthermore, after menopause, women can tend toward greater insulin resistance and lower muscle tone, especially with inadequate fitness habits. Lastly, TSH in this slightly elevated range may truly indicate an early hypothyroid pattern, as your pituitary is yelling at your thyroid gland to produce a little more. This number may be more advantageous over the age of sixty-five, but at younger ages, this level of TSH is associated with minor symptoms. If you have mild insulin resistance (HOMA-IR > 2.0), your TSH may lower following the dietary and fitness steps that improve your insulin resistance numbers. Two other reasons to have a slightly high TSH include caloric restriction (<1800 cal) or vigorous exercise in the prior twelve hours from the blood draw.

>6.0 uIU/mL: Clinically, most practitioners agree that when you have a TSH above 6.0, you will experience enough hypothyroid symptoms to warrant a more-robust medical treatment. Your health-care practitioner should be well versed in the options for thyroid prescriptions and be willing to personalize a hormonal treatment for you.

2. Thyroxine, Free (Free T4)

Optimal Range: 0.9–1.7 ng/dL (11.6–21.9 pmol/L)

T4 is a pre-hormone; it has little metabolic activity in this form compared to T3. T4 represents the production capability of your thyroid gland as nearly all the T4 measured in the blood stream was made in and released from your thyroid. T4 is made from the protein tyrosine and four iodine molecules. Nutritionally, iodine is an essential nutrient in small doses; this and other thyroid-related nutrients will be spelled out in more detail in Step Six. To activate the T4 molecule, one of the iodine molecules must be removed, thus making it the more active T3.

Your Free T4 ranges:

<0.9 ng/dL (<11.6 pmol/L): Assess your overall nutrition. Ensure adequate dietary protein because in the thyroid hormone, as the letter "T" signifies, is a protein called tyrosine. The number after the letter T stands for the number of attached iodine molecules so, as you would expect, you also need adequate nutritional iodine—*at least* 100 mcg of iodine daily. If the low FT4 is due to primary hypothyroid, you would expect to see an elevated TSH, as your pituitary gland works harder to stimulate your thyroid gland to make more T4. Early in the process of hypothyroid and low T4, your body compensates to convert more T4 to active T3, so Free T3 is often in the normal range despite low Free T4.

0.9–1.7 ng/dL (11.6-21.9 pmol/L): Normal range; your thyroid gland is adequately producing hormone in response to the TSH and feedback mechanisms.

>1.7 ng/dL (>21.9 pmol/L): This indicates excessive thyroid hormone because of an internal process or due to a medication dosage. Either way, discuss this with your health-care provider to properly evaluate for a hyperthyroid pattern, especially if you have a low TSH, a finding that confirms overactive, or hyperthyroid.

3. Triiodothyronine, Free (Free T3, FT3)

Optimal Range: 2.3–4.2 pg/mL (0.035–0.065 pmol/L)

Only a small amount of the circulating T3 was produced by your thyroid gland, and of that, only a small amount is in the unbound form, Free T3. Therefore, your Free T3 status is not regulated by your thyroid gland production; it is the activity of "de-iodinase" enzymes inside your cells. This set of enzymes turns the T3 activation on and off on an hourly basis.

You may insufficiently convert T4 into T3, or it may be an excessive conversion of active T3 to a permanently inactive form called "reverse T3" (rT3). Conditions like stress and moderate to extreme exercise cause this phenomenon, where to conserve energy, your body will "deactivate" some of your thyroid hormone. This happens more in deconditioned individuals. Like TSH, improvements in your active T3 should be seen over time when you improve other parts of your metabolism through the coming steps in the Blood Code.

Your Free T3 Ranges

<2.3 pg/mL (<0.035 pmol/L): Low and borderline low T3 with a normal T4 indicates a diminished conversion in the cells of your body, not a problem with the thyroid gland. T3 activation goes down with insulin resistance; with strenuous exercise, especially in hot temperatures; with caloric restriction; with poor conditioning; with stress . . . this list could go on. Essentially, as you take the steps toward a more balanced dietary and fitness lifestyle, and improve your insulin sensitivity and fitness, your low T3 should improve over time.

2.3–4.2 pg/mL (0.035–0.065 pmol/L): This range indicates adequate T3 activation. Free T3 fluctuates throughout the day, so variations within this normal range are expected.

>4.2 pg/mL (>0.065 pmol/L): Like elevated Free T4, discuss this with your health-care provider. Your body has evolved with a natural inclination to burn less and store more, so when the body is oddly burning more, the hyper state needs to be properly evaluated and understood.

This simple table shows the common interaction between TSH (uIU/mL), T4, and T3:

TSH	T4	T3	Interpretation
Sl High (4–6)	Normal	Normal	Insulin resistance or early / mild hypothyroidism
High (>6)	Normal	Normal	Mild hypothyroidism
High (>6)	Low	Low/normal	Hypothyroidism
Low	Normal	Normal	Mild hyperthyroidism
Low	High/normal	High/normal	Hyperthyroidism

There are more-rare conditions with the pituitary and hypothalamic release of TSH and TRH; any significant abnormality should be discussed with your health-care provider.

4. Thyroid Antibodies: Thyroid Peroxidase Antibodies (Anti-TPO, TPO Ab)

Optimal Range <30 IU/mL
S.I. units are equal numbers stated as kIU/L

A thyroid antibody called anti-thyroid peroxidase, or anti-TPO, indicates whether you are a carrier for the hypothyroid trait. This immune antibody can sit in waiting for many decades and then, after some unforeseen trigger, it might "take out" a portion of your thyroid activity. This antibody is usually present in people with a strong family history of hypothyroidism.

30–100 IU/mL: This is a slight increase from the normal range. While elevated TPO antibodies does indicate you have a greater likelihood of developing hypothyroidism, they can uneventfully sit in waiting throughout your lifetime without ever causing a problem. A positive

TPO antibody means that you are more likely to need treatment, typically with a prescription hormone, if you head toward hypothyroid numbers with your TSH, even in the slightly high 4–6 uIU/mL range.

>100 IU/mL: At this high level of antibody, you are the most likely to develop hypothyroid problems if conditions are "just right." The most common cause of primary hypothyroidism is a condition called Hashimoto's thyroiditis. Big, intimidating name, I know, but it loses its threatening nature once you understand it more. The hallmark of the condition is the presence of antibodies that target the thyroid gland (the TPO antibody) and another called the thyroglobulin antibody. Many people have elevated antibodies but never develop a thyroid condition in their lives. Here lies the evolutionary theory: The TPO antibodies sit in waiting, and if "times get tough"—low caloric intake with a chronic stress response, or perhaps a threatening immune-system trigger—the antibodies will come to life and take out some of the function of the thyroid gland to help you preserve your capital.

Slight hypothyroid activity can result in body fat that is distributed around the arms and legs. So let's hit Step Two for one more quick measurement: no blood draw, no lab— just you and your skin.

The Blood Code: Table of Units Conversion

Test Name	U.S. standard unit	Conversion Factor For U.S. to S.I. → multiply For S.I. to U.S. ← divide	Standard International (S.I.)
WBC	%	0.01	unit of 1
Hemoglobin (Hgb)	g/dL	10	g/L
Hematocrit (Hct)	%	0.01	unit of 1
BUN	mg/dL	0.357	mmol/L
Creatinine	mg/dL	88.4	umol/dL
Glucose	mg/dL	0.0556	mmol/L
Insulin	uIU/mL	6.0	pmol/L
HgbA1c	%	[%-2.15] * 10.9	mmol/mol
Triglyceride (TG)	mg/dL	0.011	mmol/L
HDL cholesterol	mg/dL	0.026	mmol/L
Total cholesterol	mg/dL	0.026	mmol/L
Ferritin	ng/mL	1	ug/L
Vitamin D	ng/mL	2.5	nmol/L
TSH	uIU/mL	1	mIU/L
Free T4	ng/dL	12.9	pmol/L
Free T3	pg/dL	0.015	pmol/L

Liver enzymes AST and ALT along with other components of the complete blood count (CBC) such as MCV, MCH and platelets are identical between systems.

HGB A1C Conversion Chart

U.S. Standard: %	S.I.: mmol/mol
4.5	26
5.0	31
5.5	36
5.7	39
5.9	41
6.1	43
6.3	45
6.5	47
7.0	53
7.5	58
8.0	64

Summarize your Blood Code results here for easy reference:

Test Date:						
Triglyceride, mg/dL						
HDL, mg/dL						
* TG:HDL ratio						
Glucose, mg/dL						
Insulin, uIU/mL						
* HOMA-IR (GxI÷405)						
HgbA1C, %						
ALT enzyme						
Vitamin D						
Ferritin						
TSH						
Free T4						
Free T3						
Other Tests:						

*For these calculations, use U.S. standard units

Step Two: Measure Yourself with Skin-Fold Calipers

The measure of who we are is what we do with what we have.
—Vince Lombardi, NFL football coach

This is an optional but instrumental step that reveals the effect of your metabolism. It's right there; you're wearing it.

You must be saying to yourself by now, "All this talk about blood tests!" Fortunately, the information that will guide you is not all hidden inside your body; some of it is expressed *on* your body, and it is waiting to be measured. You will need to get past any reservations you have about grabbing your skin and measuring the fat that lies underneath. It is no more than pinching with one hand and measuring with an easy-to-read skin-fold caliper in the other hand. The back measurement requires a buddy, but buddies come in handy for motivation too. I have taken skin-fold measurements tens of thousands of times throughout my practice, and research proves that practice makes more perfect.

If you are new to taking skin-fold measurements, you will have a little more variability in your results, but since you will be consistently measuring yourself or someone around you, you will become more consistent over time with your newfound skill. There is great value in having an at-home test that accurately measures your progress as you make dietary and fitness changes.

In my experience, I do see some patterns that are worth describing.

- Ninety-five percent of women think they are carrying all their fat at their stomachs. This may be because when you look down, you hunch forward, thereby creating abdominal rolls. Maybe it is more cultural. Whatever the reason, the fat storage is only higher in a woman's hips/abdomen about 20 percent of the time. Excess fat on the body is usually on the back, where muscles are rarely engaged, or it's on the arms, perhaps due to a sluggish thyroid pattern or lack of strength and resistance exercise. The punch line: When a good answer is a simple measurement away, why guess?

- Most teenage and young men carry excess body fat on their backs. Again, I think this is the result of a hunched posture, and can be best corrected with a well-designed, good-form fitness routine that strengthens "the backside" of the core.

- When men hit their forties, they are most likely to store the extra body fat at their hips and back. I believe that the generalized lack of fitness in a man's lifestyle is the major player here, and male hormones are a mixed blessing. Testosterone, like insulin, signals the body to make more tissue, especially on the torso. Compared to women, the male hormone balance allows men to develop significantly more muscles on their chest and back with body-building. But the hormones promote the growth of tissue, not necessarily muscle, so in the absence of adequate fitness habits, the growth of tissue will be body fat. By a man's mid-forties, they are often more sedentary in their workplace, and at the same time, a couple days of exercise per week is inadequate. The calipers don't lie. The gain in body fat measured at the hip compared to the triceps measurement is a beacon of heart disease risk.

Policy and research continues to fixate on the simplistic notion that weight gain causes illness, and weight loss reduces illness. The inconvenient truth is that weight loss does not result in less disease and a healthier life. *Fat loss does. An active lifestyle does. Promoting more insulin sensitivity does.* But weight loss as an end point does not effectively predict health and longevity. Skin-fold calipers are an inexpensive, reliable and accurate tool to measure the *amount* of body fat and mark *where* your body is storing it.

If you set a goal of weight loss, you must use calipers.

While studies have clearly found that weight loss does not add meaningful years to your life, it is a $60 billion industry in America, so I expect "weight loss" supplements and programs will continue to be marketed with abandon. People who experience weight loss with fad diets, stimulants, or during life stress, lose a significant amount of muscle and connective tissue. To add insult to injury here, when the weight is re-gained, even more fat and less muscle is put on than before the weight loss. So again, a weight scale is terribly misleading: A pound of fat is weighed equally with the stuff you don't want to lose, like muscle, connective tissue, and bone density. Calipers will show you what counts, and will help you to track your progress toward fat loss.

How to Measure

The Most Common Questions about Skin-Fold Calipers

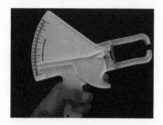

What are skin-fold calipers, and where do I get them?

Skin-fold calipers are simple devices that measure the thickness of a fold of skin and the attached tissue and fats underneath. In my practice I have often taught people how to use them. I have a $250 professional one, but prefer to use the $20 one; it's accurate and easier to read. It is available at TheBloodCode.com. Other skin-fold calipers, as long as you practice with them, will work.

Are skin-fold calipers and the resultant body fat measurement like the body mass index (BMI)?

Skin-fold calipers are a far more accurate method to assess your health status than BMI. BMI is a simple calculation of total weight compared to your height.

BMI relies on the imperfect scale which measures one thing: gravitational force upon your body on the surface of the Earth. A scale does not discern the kind of tissue creating the pressure. Fat, muscle, bone, and brain: You might want to keep some and not others. The scale will not help you to do that.

Conditioned strength athletes are considered obese on a BMI chart due to their bone and muscle density. People with low muscle mass and osteoporosis are rewarded as "lean" on the same chart. I have seen weight lifters denied their "preferred status" at a workplace wellness program due to a slightly elevated BMI despite low to normal body fat percentage. Jane Brody in the *New York Times* summarized a 2010 study on BMI accuracy, stating that BMI misclassified people 41 percent of the time. Sadly, despite being inaccurate and outdated, BMI remains a centerpiece of public health initiatives.

What about the electronic measurement of body fat?

Bioelectric impedance analyzers (BIA) are consumer-priced devices that either stand alone or are integrated into the mechanics of common bathroom scales. These devices measure skin resistance, and have substantial variability depending upon hydration, gender, race, etc. In addition to being inaccurate, these methods also do not compare and contrast different locations on your body. You will learn in this chapter that if you successfully lower your insulin, the body fat at your waist will go down. However, the body fat found on the back of your upper arm relates to your fitness habits, not diet. Electronic devices do not show you *where* the fat is.

There are laboratory-grade BIA devices used in some clinics that use four points of contact to create a more-complete measurement of electrical impedance. These high-cost devices can give you some level of accuracy provided the person is at the same hydration status from one test to the next. Unless you have several thousand dollars to spend on the high-grade devices, forget the bathroom-scale versions. Comparative studies have shown that simple skin-fold calipers in the hands of a practiced individual are as accurate as the most expensive BIA devices.[1]

How do I use my skin-fold calipers?

Video instruction and case reports can be found at TheBloodCode.com.

A skin-fold caliper is a device that measures the thickness of a fold of skin in millimeters (mm), with its underlying layer of fat. Research has shown that the thickness of this fold, at certain key locations on your body, is representative of the total amount of fat on your body. Pinch

59

with the fingers as much of the skin fold as "tissue traction" allows; firmly hold the pinch with your finger and thumb, and place the calipers next to your pinched fingers. Some people do carry a little more edema under their skin. A firm pinch, which might be tender, will push the fluid away from the point where the calipers measure. The caliper points should contact the skin right next to where your fingers are pinching firmly. To address variations in measurements, you might want to pinch three times in a row and take the lower of the three. The caliper will point to the millimeter thickness of your skin fold.

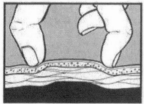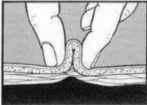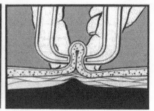

Where to Measure Body Fat

Men and women get an accurate body fat measurement by measuring four total points. Points should always be done on the same side of the body (I always use the right side). You will find that one layer of thin clothing does not substantially alter your measurement, but try to be directly on the skin when learning; it's easier. The four points are:

1) **Triceps**—midway down the back of your upper arm

2) **Biceps**—midway down the front of your upper arm

3) **Back**—under your shoulder blade, at a 35- to 45-degree downward angle

4) **Hip**—slightly forward of the top of the "hip bone," or iliac crest

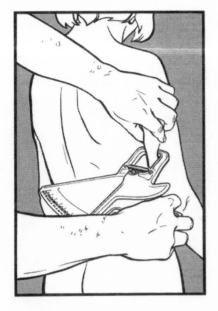

#1 Triceps location is halfway between the shoulder and elbow joints. The fold is taken in a vertical direction on the midline of the back of the upper arm.

FIGURE #1

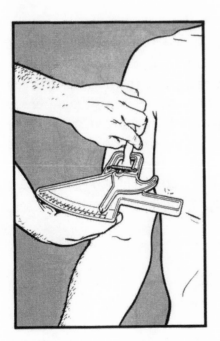

#2 Biceps measurement is taken the same way as the triceps, except it is on the midline of the front of the upper arm, midway between the elbow and the top of the shoulder.

FIGURE #2

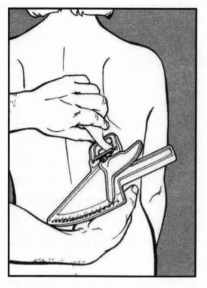

#3 Subscapular on the back: This is located just below the shoulder blade, taken at a 30- to 45-degree angle. There is an obvious band of fat here, but it might take a slight lean backward to get a good pinch. It's like a love handle under the shoulder blade.

FIGURE #3

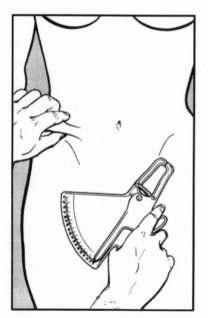

#4 Front of the hip: The measuring point on the side of the waist is taken a little toward the front, about 30 degrees from the side; this is called the "mid-axillary line." If you were to draw a line from the front crease of the armpit down to the waist, you would be at a right angle forward. It is on top of the iliac crest (hip bone), and should be approximately horizontal.

FIGURE #4

How to Interpret

Understanding Your Skin-Fold Measurements

Now that you have your skin-fold measurements for different parts of your body, you can identify your metabolic strengths and weaknesses, and unlock how to create dietary and fitness habits that will provide you with healthy progress. Each measurement is in millimeters. Together you can add them and look at the conversion chart on page 69 to get your total percentage of body fat. But before you add the skin-fold measurements to get a total, *compare the locations.* This comparison will indicate whether you need to put greater effort into your diet or your exercise habits to achieve the results you want.

Your healthy, well-conditioned goal
Hip = Triceps = Back

In millimeters, your body should have about the same amount of fat under the skin at the triceps, back, and hip area.

This means that your body is not carrying excessive fat in one location. *Having an evenly distributed amount of body fat in these areas is a mark of a balanced metabolism.* When these measurements are not near equal, the fun begins. If you found you have high insulin, you probably have a higher skin-fold reading at your hip. Long-distance runners will typically have lower body fat at the hip due to the recurrent depletion of abdominal tissue fats from extended aerobic workouts. Postmenopausal women that avoid upper body exercise will have their highest number at their triceps.

Time to grab the calipers, take your measurements, and have some fun.

<u>Your hip</u> measurement reflects your dietary trends. If body fat goes up in the hip, a shape sweetly referred to as the apple, it is usually due to excess dietary carbohydrates in your diet; conversely, if body fat on the hip drops, this is due to a reduction in stored carbohydrates. Insulin resistance and high insulin create a disproportionate increase in body fat at the hip.

Body fat goes *through* your body; it isn't just under your skin. The body fat measured under the skin with the skin-fold calipers is reflective of the fat that is stored deeper within your body in that region. Body fat on the arms and legs indicates poor fitness status; while it may be unattractive to you, it doesn't, on its own, indicate high heart disease risk, whereas body fat at the hip and torso reflects fat that has also deposited around your liver and heart area. Heart disease risk is strongly associated with excessive fat on the torso/hip region.

If the hip:triceps ratio is 2:1, in women, I strongly suspect type 2 diabetes, or at least severe insulin resistance. The Blood Code Discovery and Progress Panels can confirm this clinical suspicion. The same type 2 diabetes suspicion arises when the hip:triceps ratio is 3:1 in men.

If your caliper measurement is higher at the hip, this is the location of body fat that rightly gets the bad rap, indicating an increased risk of heart attack, stroke, dementia, some cancers—and the list goes on. If this is your trouble spot, Step Four of The Blood Code will help you to set carbohydrate limits that will reverse this trend.

<u>Your triceps</u> reflect the tone of your extremities. Your legs mirror the same pattern as your arms, so do not need to be tested separately. If your triceps is the highest number, it may be because you are "out of

shape," but people with hypothyroid can show the same imbalance. The fruit analogy describes this state as a pear. Fitness habits need to change to address this imbalance. Results are usually quick; if your body has already shown the ability to make fat, it has the hormonal ingredients to make muscle. Good fitness habits need to be put in place to effect this change.

Your back shows a combination of dietary carb balance and conditioning. In my clinical experience, your back is the most difficult body fat to reduce, due to the ubiquitous slumped posture and weak "core" that coincides with auto driving, computer keyboards, and small screens. Combine this sedentary, collapsed posture with excess dietary carbohydrates and you have a recipe for a fatty backside. In agriculture, to get a higher fat content on the back straps of livestock, you limit the animal's movement and feed it a high-carb diet with grains. This is an unhealthy environment for both livestock and humans.

Since I, for one, am not going to get rid of my technological advances, my fitness life is of primal importance. Prior to doing any exercise, make sure that you have been properly instructed to keep your core body posture upright and your shoulder blades engaged, back and down. More instruction is available at TheBloodCode. com, where we continually post instructional videos, and will have a referral list for trainers familiar with The Blood Code fitness principles.

Your bicep reflects conditioned muscle tone in the extremities. With a normal hormonal balance and muscle tone, the biceps should measure about half of the triceps. With leaner athletes, it will be even less than half the triceps. If the biceps are carrying higher proportional body fat, specific resistance and dynamic exercise of the extremities is needed.

Summary of your four possible findings:

- If skin-fold calipers measure equally in triceps, back, and hip, your diet and fitness habits are of equal importance.
- If your hip number is higher than your triceps, you are insulin-resistant, and you probably have high insulin. Carbohydrate limits will be especially important for you.
- If your triceps number is higher than your hip, your arms need more exercise and strength; if this imbalance remains persistent, your thyroid needs to be evaluated.
- If your back is highest, you are in the hunchback world of driving, texting, and typing. You need to move toward core fitness *and* lower carbs.

Take the Leap

If you discover that your body fat total is above normal, your excessive body fat is actually setting your metabolism to be *more* insulin-resistant. Here's the heartbreaker: *The more fat you have, the more fat your body will produce if nothing changes.* I know it may seem unfair, but it is the unvarnished truth. Fat begets more fat. To reverse this process, quickly and effectively, *a leap is better than baby steps.*

Why *not* baby steps? I know that other experts recommend making small, "bite-sized" changes, because, I'm afraid to say, they don't believe you can meaningfully change your habits. But I have seen thousands of similar people make the changes that free up their health and reverse disease, so I know you can do it. When you see and feel rapid improvement within a short period of time, you will more confidently stick with your new habits, and over time, there is justice. It becomes easier.

That's the good news: As your body becomes leaner over a greater surface area, insulin resistance reduces and the process reverses. A leaner, more-insulin-responsive body begets easier weight management, because the metabolic activity that promotes weight gain is no longer activated. Maintenance becomes the "easy" part of living up to your Blood Code. The steps in *The Blood Code* will help you take the leap, but it's important to realize from the outset that the dietary and fitness habits in your lifestyle are not an either-or decision; both need to be addressed in your daily life.

The location of the fat loss should steer your progress and help you decide whether to emphasize diet or exercise; measure every two to four weeks.

If your skin-fold caliper measurement gets smaller in your hip, it is due to an improvement in your diet. You are storing less abdominal body fat, probably due to your Blood Code Diet.

If your skin-fold caliper measurement gets smaller in the triceps, it is because of conditioning and better exercise. You are in better shape.

If your skin-fold calipers show proportional loss in all locations, you are doing a good job improving both your diet and exercise habits.

Chart Your Body Fat Numbers

You can add the four numbers together and use a conversion chart to get to your *total body fat percentage*. In the world of fitness and body fat assessment, a great deal of energy is spent on studies that compare the accuracy of a particular technique. The gold standard requires full body submersion into a tank that measures water displacement. Impractical, right? Calipers with well-established conversion charts are a pretty close second for accuracy, and obviously more practical. The Blood Code conversion chart is based upon the Durnin and Womersly data. Rather than having five different charts for different age groups, The Blood Code has only two charts: one for men and one for women, based upon a thirty- to fifty-year-old. If you are active and in your teens, your body fat percentage will be 1 to 2 percentage points lower than listed. If you are over sixty, your true body fat percentage might be 1 to 2 percentage points higher than listed on the conversion table. Data that tracks this trend have shown that people with the most active fitness lifestyles have total body fat percentages that reflect a much younger person; therefore, the thirty- to fifty-year-old conversion chart *is* accurate if you remain fit into your seventies and beyond.

The Blood Code Charts
Your skin-fold measurements are read off the caliper, in mm.

DATE →						
TRICEPS						
BICEPS						
BACK						
HIP						
Total mm						
Body fat %						

Don't get caught up on the total body fat percentage and apply the same angst that the scale has caused you over the years. Once again, the balance and distribution of body fat location is of greater importance.

The Blood Code Body Fat Evaluation Table

For Women		For Men	
TOTAL MM	BODY FAT %	TOTAL MM	BODY FAT %
14–15	12	12–13	7
16–17 Too Low	14	14–15 Too Low	8
18–19	15	16–17	9
20–21	17	20–21	11
22–23 Below Normal	18	22–23 Below Normal	12
24–25	19	24–25	13
26–27	20	26–27	14
28–29	21	27–28	15
30–34	22	29–31	16
35–39	23	32–35	17
40–44 Normal	25	36–38 Normal	18
45–49	26	39–42	19
50–54	28	43–45	20
55–59	29	46–49	21
60–64	30	50–54	22
65–69	31	55–59	23
70–74 Too High	32	60–65 Too High	24
75–79	33	66–73	25
80–84	34	74–79	26
85–89	35	80–85	27
90–94	36	86–91	28
95–99	37	92-98	29
100–109 Obese	38	99–105 Obese	30
110–119	39	106–115	31
120–129	40	116–125	32
130–139	41	126–135	33
140–150	42	136–145	34
151–160	43	146–156	35

Body Fat Categories and Their Meaning

Too low: Some athletes perform at this level, but they should not remain here for long. Using boxing jargon, this is called "fighting weight"—not the body fat at which you should live or train, but where you might temporarily end up on fight/race day. This category is not healthy, nor is it associated with longevity. With such low body fat, any workout that lasts longer than one hour will cause muscle breakdown, or worse. There are few to no reserves; if you experience any additional stress, you have little ability to withstand it. For example, lack of sleep, an emotionally or physically stressful event, an injury, or an underlying medical condition—any of these will result in "breakdown" very quickly due to the lack of caloric reserves and fat-soluble nutrient storage. Therefore, this category should only be an end result of extreme athletic fitness training, not a general health goal. If you are at this level of body fat, daily nutrition is critical to prevent the breakdown of your ever-important proteins. Nutrient-dense proteins and fats need to be present at all meals, and if you also have low insulin, carbohydrates should not be overly restricted. Athletes in this lean state need to ensure adequate protein intake within one hour following any workout.

Below normal: As the name implies, this category marks someone who is running a lean ship. Like a lean-running operation, though, if inflow and outflow are not properly managed, the system can break down relatively quickly. For example, if a manufacturing business runs lean, it means they have very little inventory in storage. This may be efficient, but if one part of the process is interrupted—say, a bolt (or a meal) fails to arrive on time—the whole production is compromised, because there is not sufficient inventory available to maintain good performance. To really enjoy this efficient metabolism, you will need to ensure that you maintain an optimal and balanced nutritional intake, regular meals, good sleep habits, and proper exercise. This category is what I term *conditionally normal,* and should not necessarily be a goal for you. If you are in this range, further weight loss is not your goal. Your triceps and hip measurements should be balanced.

Normal: You will see that this category has the largest range in the body fat conversion charts. Fad weight-loss programs frequently try to sell people on the "lower-is-better" theory. This is, in fact, untrue. Suffice to say that normal range, is, well . . . normal. Within this range, there is no increased risk of illness if you are in one half versus another. If your goal is to be in better shape, or you need to improve some insulin-resistance numbers from your Blood Code Panel, the changes you make in your fitness habits and diet will likely result in a lower total body fat percentage, even if you started in the normal range. But remember: Your intention should not be a trite, "lower-is-better" attitude. Family genetics play a role in your body composition; you may be at your genetic optimum at the lower half of normal, while others will reach their goal at the upper half of normal. Balance between the skin-fold locations, optimal blood test results, and great fitness are all attainable within this category. Most people will live at their healthiest within this range.

Above normal: This category shows that you have plenty of reserves. To use the manufacturing analogy, your body is cluttered with parts, and excess inventory is lying around in boxes. This burdensome inventory is part of an inefficient system, and corporations are taxed on this excess at year end. In your body, the inventory is the excess fat deposits, and your taxes are a future illness or injury. Above normal may not be much actual weight on a scale, but chronic disease risks start to show up here: elevated blood pressure, high triglyceride:HDL ratio, and elevated fasting blood sugar are all markers of increased heart disease, cancer, and dementia risk. Above normal is your time to act before the trend continues. The steps that follow will help you to better utilize the pantry of calories that you are wearing on your body.

Obese: This is the category that is conclusively linked to compromised health and long-term illness. Across the board, people don't feel good in this category, whether it's physically or emotionally. The reality of this category shows little pity. As body fat percentage increases, greater insulin resistance occurs and lower basal metabolic rates are measured, resulting in a continual progression. Everyone in this category will need to exercise to compensate for the slow resting metabolic rate that results from higher body fat stores. As a rule, once in the obese category, you have to be more active than someone with lower body fat in order to burn the same amount of energy. In addition, body fat is more insulin-resistant than muscle, so once you're in this category, carbohydrates cause even more fat storage and blood sugar problems than when you become leaner. Strong emphasis on the Blood Code Diet with carbohydrate restriction is imperative to change this insulin-resistant trend. A leap is a good start; make some big changes in your daily habits. The following steps offer you the ability to apply self-directed changes that will move you in the right direction.

Skin-fold calipers measure the end result of your daily metabolism—the calories that you wear on your body in the form of tissue fat. It is time to put this together with your Blood Code Panel results and find the right steps for you to unlock your personal Blood Code.

Review the Basics:

The absolute number measured by calipers, in millimeters, should be similar between the triceps, back, and hip.

Triceps = Back = Hip

If triceps measure higher than the hip, it implies a relative lack of muscle tone or slower metabolism. In this case, it's important to perform a thorough thyroid panel and address your fitness habits to provide strenuous exercise (see Step Four).

If your back measures higher than hip or triceps, it implies poor core muscle tone or excess carbohydrates in your diet. It is imperative to exercise in a posture that engages your back and core, and your carbohydrate intake likely needs to be reduced.

If your hip measures higher than your back or triceps, correct your carbohydrate intake, first and foremost. Not only do you have some insulin resistance, but you are also producing a lot of extra insulin. You will likely respond quickest to dietary carbohydrate control.

Step Three: Putting It All Together—IR, High Insulin, Hypothyroid

"Are these the shadows of things that will be, or are they the shadows of things that may be only?"
[Scrooge insists urgently] "These events can be changed. A life can be made right."
—Charles Dickens, *A Christmas Carol* (Scrooge's monologue with the Ghost of Christmas Future)

You have been introduced to the measurements that plot your current metabolism. Before I describe the steps that will unlock your personalized diet, nutrition, and fitness program, I'd like to help you see how your blood test results and skin-fold measurements fit together, and how your lifestyle habits are likely to impact your success. A metaphor might be useful to help understand your metabolic strength and efficiency: Enter the automobile.

Car Models and Your Metabolic Code

I will say it again: Insulin resistance and mild hypothyroid are not, by nature, bad, and should not be considered diseases. In fact, these traits have certain strengths; for example, a large, heavy vehicle with a huge gas tank is perfect for the job of hauling heavy material long distances. It just doesn't make a good driving-around-town car. Let's use this metaphor to describe the different metabolic efficiencies and inefficiencies that describe your metabolism.

Two Types of Insulin Resistance

Insulin resistance comes in two different models: *high insulin* and *normal insulin*. In the real world, there are variations that mix elements of the two models, but the two archetypes provide a helpful comparison of the two expressions of insulin resistance.

High insulin (sport utility oversize XL): This car has an extra big gas tank, and it is full to the rim. There are also jugs of extra fuel in the trunk, a couple on the backseat, and maybe even one more in the front passenger seat. Now that I describe it, this car sounds downright dangerous, but perfect for a hauling a heavy load a long, long distance without having to stop for refueling.

The large gas tank is your oversize liver, and the fuel canisters represent the excessive glycogen and fat on and in your body. Triglycerides are usually high (TG>150) in your bloodstream, and your skin-fold calipers measure higher on your hip than on your triceps. All this extra fat is like having extra fuel tanks in the passenger seat. This is great if you need to go a couple thousand miles before the next fueling station, but realistically, your body's next fuel stop probably comes within hours, not weeks.

Normal (or low) insulin (fuel-efficient sedan with always-full tank): In this car, there is a normal-size gas tank, but it goes a remarkably long way before running out of fuel. The effect of insulin resistance is seen when driven. This car has a magical ability to use almost no fuel if driven efficiently. Driven without much stress to the engine, this car will always have enough fuel to start, and to get you around town without frequent stops for fuel. But if you reflexively fill the tank with gasoline every hundred miles, you will create a dangerous overflow of gasoline.

The glucose and carbohydrates in your diet are the fuel in the gas tank. Over the course of a day, the low-insulin model will have blood sugars above normal, unless there is some strenuous exertion. Eating extra carbs when the sugar is already high is like topping off the tank to the point where the gas overflows and runs down the side of the car, and into the trunk. Dangerous, right? But instead of fuel spilling on the ground, the extra blood sugar problematically overflows into your bloodstream, body tissues, and brain. Unlike the big, high-insulin model vehicle, this normal-insulin, superefficient car model includes the 40 percent of people who develop type 2 diabetes that are *not* overweight.[1] A recent study in China galvanized this little truth. When 99,000 Chinese adults were tested, over half were prediabetic, and the vast majority of those with insulin resistance were of normal weight.[2]

Once the tank of glucose in your bloodstream is filled, you can prevent the overflow by reducing the carb intake. But what about the glucose that is already there? You can address this by exercising *inefficiently*, moving yourself as you would while driving in the city: lots of stop-and-go acceleration. This is called *interval training*, and the Fitness Principles in Step Five will spell out how to best incorporate this in your own life, according to your unique metabolism (page 159).

Allow me to extend the auto analogy to a mildly hypothyroid metabolism.

Hypothyroid and Your Car's Idle Speed

Years ago, I brought my old Volvo to an auto shop where the mechanic worked on a disproportionate number of high-mileage cars. I noticed that he adjusted the idle speed to a steady 800 rpm rather than the customary 1,000 rpm. (A note of apology to any auto mechanics who are reading this oversimplified analogy; I'm sure there's a great deal more to how a car is tuned and adjusted!)

This minor downward adjustment allows the car to work less while idling. Once the gas pedal is engaged, the acceleration of the engine is the same as it would be for a car with a higher idle speed. The lower and more-efficient idle speed, theoretically, helped allow my car to live a longer life (it's still running, in fact). Blood tests that show a TSH level >3 but <6 uIU/mL are associated with longevity. This mildly elevated TSH is loosely termed *mild hypothyroid.*

If you have been told that you have "mild hypothyroid" (TSH between 2.5 and 6), or if you medically treat hypothyroidism with hormone medications, you need to actively get your body above idle speed. If you live your life at or near your slow idle speed, you will feel sluggish and will be out of shape; your triceps measurement on skin-fold calipers will be higher than your hip. You need to rev up your engine speed before functioning in your day.

If you tend toward a mild hypothyroid state, your day will go better with morning exercise to warm up your metabolism, and some strenuous fitness to get the muscles toned in your arms and legs. Idle speed is only when your body is at complete rest. Just like the low-idle car, once you are physically active, the gas pedal of fitness metabolically heats up your body, making your initial idle speed moot.

Nondiabetic conditions when you have, and are ignoring, insulin resistance:
Abdominal fat gain
Essential hypertension
Lipid abnormalities
Polycystic ovary syndrome
Nonalcoholic fatty liver disease

Clinical conditions that can be the first signs of insulin resistance:
Psoriasis
Gout
Restless leg syndrome / muscle cramps
Erectile dysfunction
Depression
Sleep apnea
Androgenic alopecia (baldness)
Dementia
Swollen joints that are not improved with typical treatment

Too much of a good thing can be too much, of course, so if your idle speed is too low (TSH >5–6 mIU/mL), your car will sputter and stall while at idle, especially in cold weather. This level of hypothyroidism should be medically corrected for most people. Again, even with a hormonal prescription, you need to drive your body with a bit more on the gas pedal of exercise, especially in the morning.

Your blood tests and skin-fold measurements provide a viewing window into the metabolic events that occur in your body. This is what you will see:

- Whether or not you currently express insulin resistance
- Whether you have high insulin
- Whether you tend toward mild hypothyroid, or high TSH

This discussion would be useless if there was no way to turn it around and move toward your metabolic recovery and insulin sensitivity. By the end of this chapter you will be able to gauge how insulin-resistant you are, and whether a slower thyroid is interfering with your metabolism. You will then be able to self-direct your dietary/carbohydrate, nutritional, and fitness habits that are specific for your body.

As presented in Step One, the test result ranges below will first list the U.S. standard unit followed by the S.I. international unit in parentheses. The conversion chart is found on page 53.

Are You Insulin Resistant?

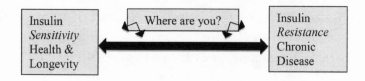

You show no insulin resistance if your Blood Code reveals:

- Fasting glucose is between 75–95 mg/dL (4.2–5.3 mmol/L).
- TG:HDL ratio is near 1.0, +/- 0.5.
- Fasting insulin is between 3–8 uIU/mL (18–48 pmol/L).
- HgbA1C level is less than 5.6% (<37 mmol/mol).
- Glucose/insulin as HOMA-IR is near 1 (.5–1.5).
- Your total body fat is <28% for men and <32% for women.

You show slight insulin resistance if you have two or more of the following:

- Fasting glucose is greater than 95 mg/dL (5.3 mmol/L).
- TG:HDL ratio is greater than 2.
- Fasting insulin is greater than 8 uIU/mL (>48 pmol/L).
- HgbA1C level is greater than 5.5% (>36 mmol/mol).
- HOMA-IR is greater than 1.5.
- The skin fold at your hip is greater than that at your triceps (by at least 5 mm).

You show moderate insulin resistance if you have three or more of the following:

- Fasting glucose is greater than 100 mg/dL (>5.6 mmol/L).
- TG:HDL ratio is 3 or greater.
- Fasting insulin is greater than 10 uIU/mL (>60 pmol/L).

- HgbA1C level is greater than 5.7% (>39 mmol/mol).
- HOMA-IR is greater than 2.5.
- The skin fold at your hip measures near twice that at your triceps.

You show severe insulin resistance if you have three or more of the following:

- Fasting glucose is greater than 110 mg/dL (>6.1 mmol/L). Greater than 125 mg/dL (>7.0 mmol/L) is diabetes.*
- TG:HDL ratio is greater than 4.
- Fasting insulin is greater than 12 uIU/mL (>72 pmol/L).
- HgbA1C level is greater than 6.0% (>42 mmol/mol). Greater than 6.4% (>46 mmol/mol) is diagnostic of diabetes.*
- HOMA-IR is greater than 3.
- The skin fold at your hip measures over twice that at your triceps.

If you have a diagnosis of type 2 diabetes, it also means that you currently express severe insulin resistance.

Insulin Resistance: What It Really Means for You

Over 40 percent of Americans are currently insulin-resistant, and the majority will develop type 2 diabetes in their lifetime given the current trends in diet and lifestyle. Insulin resistance is a practical human characteristic rather than a disease. Even natural medicine and functional medicine advocates wrongly blame insulin resistance for hypertension, elevated lipids, fatty liver, weight gain, and diabetes.

Genetics research confirms that insulin resistance is an advantage.

Your body is designed to survive periods with few calories and great physical effort. As of early 2013, at least 15 of your 23 genes are known to carry traits related to insulin resistance, and over 30 gene locations have been confirmed to raise susceptibility to insulin resistance and higher blood sugars. *This is no mistake!*

If you like this kind of genetic analysis, the human genome and associated illnesses are cataloged with Johns Hopkins University (http://www.omim.org/entry/125853?search=t2dm &highlight=t2dm).

Insulin resistance is the metabolic force behind the term *metabolic syndrome*. Metabolic syndrome is the gray area of symptoms that lie between normal blood sugar and type 2 diabetes. Nicknames include syndrome X, prediabetes, and Reaven's syndrome. If you have insulin resistance *without high insulin,* you won't have the tendency to get very fat, but you will see a consistent rise in blood sugars over time.

In truth, insulin resistance is your perfect expression of an efficient calorie economy; inappropriate lifestyle habits are the "disease," not you. Your life habits need to be in accordance with your genetic expression.

I appreciate how difficult it is to see a positive aspect of the traits behind type 2 diabetes, a condition that is clouded by the one-sided headlines that negatively fixate on the end-stage disease in overmedicated or uncontrolled type 2 diabetics. If I hadn't seen thousands of people effectively turn their insulin resistance around—reversing weight problems, high blood pressure, lipid abnormalities, low energy, *and* type 2 diabetes—I, too, might lack the confidence and positive attitude that I maintain toward insulin resistance.

Insulin resistance is an efficiency, and is beautifully adapted to a world of outer inefficiency and effort. If you discover that you express this trait, you need to eat and exercise like the world is still a physically demanding place: no eating between meals, limited carbohydrate intake, and strenuous fitness activity.

Insulin resistance (IR) is simply when your body leaves extra glucose in the bloodstream at baseline and after meals. Hormonal, neurochemical, and anatomical processes drive IR; therefore, if you want to resolve it, you have to come at it from several different directions. I will say again: This condition does not lend itself to reductionist, pills-for-your-problems medical care. Diet, exercise, and nutrition must all be at the center of your program.

Insulin Resistance and the Action Steps Ahead of You

Step Four is dedicated to the dietary changes ahead of you; here's your chance to see what is coming. You have discovered your level of insulin resistance; now, find your carbohydrate tolerance. Let's call this your *carbohydrate code*.

Unlock your carbohydrate code per meal:

Without insulin resistance:
Breakfast: 30–40 grams
Lunch: 50–80 grams
Dinner: 50–80 grams
*TOTAL: 130–200 grams (about 550–800 calories)

Slight insulin resistance:
Breakfast: 15–25 grams
Lunch: 40–65 grams
Dinner: 40–65 grams
*TOTAL: 100–150 grams (about 400–600 calories)

Moderate insulin resistance:
Breakfast: 10–20 grams
Lunch: 20–40 grams
Dinner: 20–40 grams
*TOTAL: 50–90 grams (about 200–400 calories)

Severe insulin resistance:
Breakfast: 5–10 grams
Lunch: 10–15 grams
Dinner: 10–15 grams
*TOTAL: 25–40 grams (about 100–200 calories)

* These gram ranges are based upon a diet of about 2,000 to 2,800 calories—a dietary intake that is an ideal average for most of us. If you are an athlete and exercise more than 60 to 90 minutes daily, your carbs, fat, and proteins all need to be appropriately adjusted upward.

Step Five describes how to exercise so that you can tap into the storage tank of fats and sugars in your body. With insulin resistance, you do not just have high sugars in your bloodstream; you also have extra stored sugars in your liver, tissues, and muscles. If left to sit there, this extra sugar promotes inflammation and disease, so you need to actively clear it out. The encouraging word I can give you is that *any* exercise lowers your blood sugar; however, once your body has begun to express IR, gentle aerobic exercise will not help you turn this condition around.

Without insulin resistance: Incorporate the Four Fitness Principles at least two to three days per week. On the other days, any aerobic activity will do. Total: no less than 30 minutes.

Slight insulin resistance: Fitness Principle #2 becomes important at this stage; strenuous exercise sort of "wrings out" the muscles to utilize the stored sugar and glycogen that efficiently stores in your muscles. This should be at least every other day. On the other three days per week, general aerobic exercise is adequate, but should be a little more like the "interval training" that will be described later (see page 163).

Moderate and severe insulin resistance: Five to seven days per week, you need some strenuous exercise, even if it is for only 5 to 10 minutes; do something a few times daily. You need to use your body as if the world is the physically demanding place for which you are acclimated.

Step Six describes how nutrients such as vitamin D, when deficient, make insulin resistance worse. Furthermore, when you are insulin-resistant, you become more deficient in certain nutrients, such as magnesium. If you have insulin resistance, you are likely to have several nutrient deficiencies that make your condition worse. To fully correct your metabolism to its sweet spot, you will need to ensure that you are not deficient in several core nutrients. The more severe your insulin resistance, the greater the need to actively prevent nutrient deficiency.

I had an inquisitive patient once ask me, "If I'm insulin-resistant, why do I keep producing so much body fat?" The answer involves seeing insulin as the most skilled, primary—but not the only, worker in the business of building and storing fat. Your body works, at all costs, to avoid the damaging effect of chronically high blood sugar. Therefore, even with insulin resistance, other mechanisms will continue to turn sugar into fat and store it. Once you become more sensitive to insulin again, it's like having the star player back on your team—you'll perform better.

What does insulin resistance *feel* like? In my clinical practice I see cases of insulin resistance every day, and sometimes a person just has a good way of talking about it. Mark is just that kind of person. He was gaining fat around his waist, but came to the office for other reasons. Years later I shared before and after pictures that I had taken, and he was stunned. He hopes that his story can shed light on the health gains you can experience when you truly resolve insulin resistance.

A Case of Insulin Resistance / Metabolic Syndrome

Mark S., thirty-five years old

Mark came into my office not because of his weight, but because of a concern for his health. He knew something wasn't right. He implemented his diet change starting in March, and the September test was at six months. Mark has generously agreed to share his story in his own words (see testimonial below, on page 86; additional cases can be found on TheBloodCode website).

Panel test date	1/4/08	9/18/08
Cholesterol, mg/dL	226	208
Triglyceride, mg/dL	176	64
HDL, mg/dL	49	44
TG:HDL ratio	3.5	1.4
Fasting glucose, mg/dL	112	98
Fasting insulin, uIU/mL	13.4	—
HOMA–IR	3.7	

Date →	1/8/08	4/29/08	7/17/08	9/23/08
Triceps, mm	24	21	16	13
Biceps, mm	12	10	12	10
Back, mm	26	20	15	16
Hip, mm	43	29	24	21
Total mm	106	80	67	60
Body fat %	29%	26%	23%	22%

Mark fell into Severe IR (but not type 2 diabetes); after six months, he was in the "slight IR" category, with room to keep improving.

Skin-fold caliper measurements: Mark waited a full nine months between blood tests, but his metabolic improvement was evident in his skinfold calipers.

June 26, 2013—Owls Head, Maine

I met Dr. Richard Maurer in 2008. I was ashamed to ask for help and counsel, but I was overweight, stressed out, and very concerned about my health. Dr. Maurer immediately set me at ease, treated me with great respect, and suggested a simple blood test before he made any recommendations.

After the blood test was complete, Dr. Maurer suggested a few simple modifications to my diet. I took his advice and counsel to heart, and committed the next eight weeks to his protocol. The results were beyond amazing; they were life-changing.

The color came back into my face and skin. The red in my eyes cleared up, and I was told they sparkled. The texture of my hair changed. I slept through the night without interruption.

The things in my life that cause stress did not change, but my ability to handle stress and let it slip away changed in a big way.

On top of that, I lost tons of useless body fat.

But more importantly, my health and wellness improved a hundredfold. I became inspired and excited about my life and health.

I don't like to give people advice on their health and wellness, nor am I qualified to do so. But when people sincerely want to know how my health improved so dramatically, I refer them to Dr. Maurer, his work, and The Blood Code.

—Mark S.

Hypoglycemia

Your body has dozens of ways to prevent low blood sugar, but for short periods of time, you can experience something called *reactive hypoglycemia*. This is when your body is hyperreactive to the message of insulin after imbalanced meals. A high-carb/low-fat meal results in a burst of insulin that causes a sudden drop in blood glucose in some people. The hypoglycemia that results will be quickly remedied by a release of adrenaline and other compensatory hormones, but this reactive process doesn't feel good. This process occurs early in someone's lifetime (before age twenty-five), before any insulin resistance has set in. If you experienced reactive hypoglycemia when young, you may tend more toward IR when older (>45 years old).

When teenagers or younger children experience migraine headaches, light-headedness, hyperactivity, or inability to concentrate, insulin-reactive hypoglycemia is suspected, and the triggers for insulin, like excess carbs in the diet, should be controlled.

High Insulin: >10 uIU/mL (>70 pmol/L) and the Action

Steps Ahead of You

High insulin is a variation on insulin resistance. It causes the high TG and excess fat deposits around your middle, measurable by skin-fold calipers. In the prior section I emphasized the benefits that come with insulin resistance. Let's define what is happening with high insulin. This discussion will allow you to more fully recognize *why* your body is performing the way it is, and help lead you toward *what* you can do about it.

Insulin is an anabolic (builds tissue) hormone made in the pancreas and secreted directly into the bloodstream, in response to several different stimuli, especially the carbohydrate and protein content of a meal. Insulin replaces the storage sugar/glycogen and fat into the fuel tanks of your body—the cells of your fat, muscles, liver, etc.

> *Glucose* is the cash in your hands.
> *Glycogen* is the cash deep in your pocket.
> *Body fat* and *triglycerides* are the funds stuck in
> your bank account.

Early-stage high insulin: As you begin to secrete extra insulin, your body will take sugars from your bloodstream and turn them into fats and proteins and put them away. At this early stage, your blood sugar will usually be normal, as the glucose is turned into a better storage form: triglycerides (TG). Your TG will start to rise on your blood tests (>100 mg/dL, or >1.1 mmol/L), and you will be able to measure that fat with skin-fold calipers—specifically, your body fat measurement will be higher on your hip and back compared to your triceps. At a very young age, late teens to early twenties, you might benefit from insulin's night job: It helps your body to replenish glycogen, utilize proteins, and make muscle tissue. High insulin is actually useful for a strength-oriented athlete . . . to a point. High insulin, if let go for years, will cause your body to "numb out" and ignore the noise of insulin's message. This is the transition from insulin sensitivity to insulin resistance, and it will typically show up when you are in your forties, if not sooner.

The industry-sponsored recommendation to consume sugar-laden chocolate milk following activity is fundamentally wrong if you have the innate ability to secrete high levels of insulin naturally. Instead of the carb-heavy 3:1 ratio in chocolate milk, plain whole yogurt has closer to the desirable 1:1 ratio of carb to protein.

Late-stage high insulin: As your insulin stays high for many years, you will accumulate the effects: Triglycerides are stored everywhere. Your skin-fold caliper measurements will display excess fat storage on your hip and back; your torso is storing fat for the "big event." The organs inside the torso will also store extra fat. Your liver will have higher fat storage, causing fatty liver and elevated liver enzymes, especially the ALT enzyme. TG on the blood test will be high, above 150 mg/dL (1.7 mmol/L), and your liver will be so bogged down with fat that the "good cholesterol" can't be produced, so the HDL is low. This trend is best displayed through the TG:HDL ratio, which will be above 3.0 at this stage.

High insulin will cause a fatty torso—what we call the "apple-shaped" person. If you store significant weight around your middle, you probably have high insulin. The obesity is not your problem; the underlying insulin is the driving force. It helps to realize that insulin is insatiable: The more fat you store, the better your body will store fat. On the surface, the problem appears progressive. High insulin is remarkably misunderstood; medical headlines repeatedly "blame" obesity as the curse or underlying cause of "coronary heart disease, ischemic stroke, hypertension, dyslipidemia, type 2 diabetes, joint disease, cancer, sleep apnea, asthma, and other chronic conditions."[3] The obesity is not the horse pulling the cart; the high insulin is pulling the cart, and if left uncorrected, it will lead to subsequent insulin resistance / high blood sugar results.

Insulin Is a Gift, Not a Curse

Migratory ducks and fatty liver. Pardon me for comparing you to a duck, but the physiology is similar. Ducks in my home state of Maine spend September gorging on the late-summer wild rice in the freshwater marshes. This behavior creates a disproportionately big liver in these very small teal ducks. By early October, they launch into the air and fly for more than a thousand miles without another bite of food during their journey.

Temporary fatty liver is desirable for this lifestyle; a problem only arises if the duck decides to lie around in a climate-controlled house for the next twelve months. If you have high insulin, your inner duck must not gorge on carbs and remain sedentary in a climate-controlled house and workplace.

Good news! If you have high insulin, you are the most likely among your peers to experience a rapid and dramatic improvement in your weight and metabolism with The Blood Code. Stay within your pre-scribed carbohydrate restriction and follow the fitness guidelines that reinforce strenuous, full-body workouts on an empty stomach. You do not need to carbo-load . . . ever. You already store calories exceedingly well without the extra carbo load. Measure with your skin-fold calipers every three to four weeks; you will be impressed with how quickly you improve. Step Four will be your most important intervention. Here is a bit of a preview:

Primary Dietary Steps If You Have High Insulin

Several foods and food combinations do a tremendous job of triggering a release of insulin. If you know you tend toward high insulin normally, these foods and combinations need to be carefully limited.

1) **Unfavorable carbohydrates** cause a rapid increase to your blood sugar; both simple and complex sugars are implicated.

2) **Dietary protein** has a less-pronounced effect on insulin; any meal with greater than 20 grams of protein will trigger an insulin release. Your protein choices need to be eaten with plenty of fats, not extra carbs.

3) **Stretching the stomach:** Oversized meals and volume foods trigger a stomach-stretch response, part of a neat system whereby your digestive tract lining is an endocrine gland. Your gut releases two hormones, collectively known as *incretins:* GLP-1 and GIP. These hormones stimulate insulin to help lower glucose.

4) **Combinations add up:** "Two bads equal a worse." Simple sugars when mixed with protein or complex carbs trigger a huge insulin release. While not many of you would put sugar on a steak, you probably don't hesitate when it comes to putting ketchup on a hamburger with a bun. Foods with protein, sugar, and no fiber, like ice cream and chocolate milk, are disastrous. Sugar added to bread is another ubiquitous combination, such as toast and jam, cookies, muffins, etc.

More detailed information and research about the disease risks of a lifetime of excessive insulin can be found in the "Digging Deeper" chapter.

A Case of Early High Insulin
Kevin T., twenty-one years old

Kevin was in his final year of college, and had put on weight. He felt worse after eating and suspected a food allergy. Kevin had part of his problem right: He was reacting poorly to foods, but it wasn't an allergy; it was carbs. He improved in ninety days.

Panel test date	9/1/12	12/10/12
Cholesterol, mg/dL	194	190
Triglyceride, mg/dL	196	92
HDL, mg/dL	39	52
TG:HDL	5.0	1.7
Fasting glucose, mg/dL	85	82
Fasting insulin, uIU/mL	24	12
HOMA–IR	5.0	2.4

Skin-Fold Caliper Measurements

DATE →	9/1/12	12/10/12
Triceps	12*	12
Biceps	6	5
Back	20	18
Hip	24*	14
Total mm	62	49
Body fat %	24%	21%

* High hip:triceps ratio indicates high insulin. Still in his youth, he wasn't yet unhealthy or obese.

<u>Initial Plan:</u> Carb limits: 20 grams at breakfast / 20–40 grams at lunch and dinner. Only minor exercise changes were made.

Great improvement occurred: TG:HDL and HOMA-IR are heading toward 1:1, with room to improve with a bit more strenuous and frequent exercise.

Hypothyroid, Slightly Elevated TSH, and Thyroid Antibodies

Your thyroid function represents one part of a brilliant orchestra of hormones with which your body regulates the amount of energy burned at rest. By lowering the cellular activity, you burn slightly less calories and produce a little less heat. At rest, this is referred to as a *slow or low basal metabolic rate*. You can see why this gland could become the scapegoat for all kinds of "sluggish" or weight-related symptoms.

Your thyroid panel can display several imbalances that require attention to your nutritional and fitness habits. This is not a replacement for medical advice about thyroid hormone prescriptions. The common blood test variants and subsequent action you require are listed here.

TSH is high-normal (2.5–4.0 uIU/mL), with normal T4 and T3

TSH is the most common hormone used clinically to detect early stages of a hypothyroid tendency. Research has consistently shown a link between TSH in the upper-normal range and heart disease risk.[4] But researchers are guilty of mistakenly labeling people with high-normal TSH as *mild, or subclinical, hypothyroid,* and some members of the medical community have subsequently become overzealous when it comes to dispensing thyroid prescriptions. The high-normal TSH is a case of mistaken identity; slightly high/normal TSH may not be hypothyroid at all. More-recent research has clarified that the suspicious heart disease risk associated with TSH between 2 and 4 was due primarily to underlying insulin resistance.[5] Furthermore, the insulin resistance appears to "cause" TSH to rise slightly.[6]

So, first things first: Check to see if you if you do have any other markers of insulin resistance.

Blood tests such as:
     A1C >5.6% (>37mmol/mol)
     HOMA-IR>2.5
     TG:HDL>2.5

Total body fat percentage:
>31% in women
>25% men

If your TSH is slightly elevated *and* you display insulin resistance (IR), follow the steps to correct your IR. It might improve your next TSH test.

TSH is slightly high (4–6 uIU/mL), with normal to low T4 and T3

This pattern is on the continuum of hypothyroidism. As T4 and T3 go below normal and TSH goes higher, hypothyroidism is more evident. Ultimately, the use of a thyroid hormone prescription is up to you and your health-care provider, but here are some things you must consider in order to individualize your care.

Age and hypothyroid: Hormonal activity, thyroid included, tends to be lower in people over the age of sixty-five to seventy. While some think that this thyroid decline is a reason to consider prescription thyroid hormones to combat the effects of aging, convincing animal and human studies link this natural hormonal drop with longevity.[7] TSH in large-scale studies was associated with longevity up to a level of about 8 uIU/mL; above that, and the hypothyroidism was too much of a problem.[8] As you age, your body apparently has a little more reason to preserve capital; your resting metabolism will therefore slow down slightly. If you want a bit more pep as you age, you need to place an extra degree of importance on exercise in your daily life.

Exercise and hypothyroid: Stressful exercise in less-conditioned individuals lowers the T4 and T3 thyroid hormones compared to those who are in better shape.[9] This doesn't mean you should avoid stressful exercise; on the contrary, it indicates that you should strive to be in better condition overall, so that stressful situations do not excessively reduce your thyroid activity. Extended periods of exercise—over 30 minutes, especially in a hot environment—replaces the need for some of your thyroid activity, so it is natural to have reduced thyroid hormone activity after these circumstances.[10]

Dieting and hypothyroid: Long-term low caloric intake, 1,800 calories or less, results in less thyroid hormone activity and higher TSH levels.[11] A sudden drop in caloric intake can generate a compensatory short-term drop in thyroid activity a well.

Hypothyroid as Helpful?

Some hypothyroid tendency is likely a historically advantageous adaptation, which allowed people to use fewer calories at rest, thereby squandering less precious ingested calories. Sudden strenuous exercise and decreased caloric intake both lower thyroid activity. Historically, this helped people to survive during periods of excess physical exertion and minimal food, like having to walk a long distance to get to a displaced food supply. Got it? Vigorous exercise and low caloric intake both lower your thyroid activity. All those programs that tout calorie-restrictive diets with simultaneous boot camp–style exercise will contrarily *slow* your resting metabolism. This may blow the minds of those who are thinking that the only way to drop serious weight is to train hard and reduce calories, but if you tend toward any degree of hypothyroid, your success will only be short-term, if achieved at all. The slower resting metabolism that results will only make it harder for you to maintain whatever weight loss occurred.

If you have high TSH, mild hypothyroid, or are currently being treated for hypothyroid, you will need to build very consistent dietary, nutritional, and fitness habits. Yes, even if you are treated with a thyroid hormone, the pill is not the end of your metabolic imbalance. Your hypothyroid tendency is still present at your tissues, so the lifestyle habits are critical, whether or not natural or synthetic hormonal treatment is in place.

Action Steps for Hypothyroid

Step Four dietary habits for hypothyroid must be consistent! The feast-or-famine approach will not work for your diet. You can't eat less before a vacation so that you can indulge while away. Each time you significantly reduce your caloric intake, your metabolism will quickly and efficiently compensate by slowing your resting caloric burn rate. Therefore, your total caloric intake should be relatively consistent over time. Of course, if you learn that you also express insulin resistance, you must find the carbohydrate range that is right for you and your Blood Code.

Cruciferous vegetables and hypothyroid: There are certain foods that have tremendous anti-cancer properties and are loaded with health-ful nutrients, but contain a compound that can have a subtle effect on thyroid metabolism. They are given the name *goitrogens,* and include cruciferous vegetables such as broccoli, cauliflower, Brussels sprouts, bok choy, broccolini, Chinese cabbage, kale, kohlrabi, radish, collard greens, and turnips. Many online resources exaggerate the adverse thyroid effects from these foods. People with iodine deficiency or significant hypothyroidism appear to be the only ones affected by very high doses of these raw cruciferous vegetables. But even consuming a serving of these foods daily is not enough to have the said adverse effect. Furthermore, cooking effectively inactivates their goitrogenic activity—a reason to question the fad of "juicing" for general health. In my clinical practice, I have never recommended that anyone avoid these healthful vegetables in their diet. The vegetables should be properly cooked, and you should ensure that you are not overtly deficient in the mineral iodine.

There are goitrogenic compounds in soy products, peanuts, lima beans and millet that *do not* break down with cooking like the above vegetables. Therefore, if you have thyroid tests that are outside of healthy ranges, these foods are best limited or avoided.[12]

Step Five fitness rules for hypothyroid—daily in the morning! You must exercise every day; that is first and foremost. One more time: *daily.* Your resting metabolism is a little slower with hypothyroid, but that does not carry over to your active metabolism. In fact, the metabolic effect of very strenuous exercise that lasts 45 minutes effectively replaces significant thyroid hormone activity for over 12 hours.[13] Overnight, all people experience a drop in body temperature while sleeping; those with a hypothyroid tendency require physical activity to quickly generate heat and kick-start their metabolism to normal. This does not need to take much time; a workout of 10 to 15 minutes first thing in the morning is a critical step for you to feel better throughout your day. Once you feel like the activity is heating you up, you've done enough.

Step Six nutrition guidelines for hypothyroid: The T4 hormone requires the nutrient iodine—not much, 100 to 300 mcg is considered a healthy *minimum* range. The enzymes that convert inactive T4 to the active hormone T3 are made from the mineral selenium, and require zinc to function. Low vitamin D can make hypothyroid symptoms worse. Iodine, selenium, zinc, vitamin D: all require special attention and possible supplementation to assure you avoid any deficiency that could aggravate hypothyroidism.

A Case of Hypothyroid *with* Insulin Resistance
Tony C., forty-seven years old

In 2011 Tony said succinctly, "I suspect there is some imbalance that's causing very low energy, but when I regularly exercise, I feel better."

Panel Test Date	4/27/11	3/30/12	9/7/12
Cholesterol, mg/dL	217	227	208
Triglyceride, mg/dL	175	143	84
HDL, mg/dL	43	49	50
TG:HDL	4.1	2.9*	1.7**
Glucose, fast. mg/dL	101	103*	82**
Insulin, fast. uIU/mL	7.1		5.5
TSH, uIU/mL	4.4	1.5	1.8
Vitamin D, ng/mL	15	19*	30

Skin-Fold Caliper Measurements

DATE →	4/19/11	12/10/12	9/2/12**
Triceps, mm	8	10	8
Biceps, mm	5	6	5
Back, mm	20	18	14
Hip, mm	20	16	12**
Total in mm	53	50	38
Body fat %	22%	22%	18%

* Like many people with hypothyroid, he had insulin resistance (IR), too. By 3/30/12, the thyroid prescription had corrected the TSH, but not his IR.

** Tony was able to pull his blood tests, body fat, and TG:HDL into his healthy range only after adopting a trainer-inspired fitness routine in conjunction with prescription thyroid.

High Thyroid Peroxidase (TPO>100 IU/mL)

As discussed in Step One, high TPO indicates that your immune system is at the ready, or has already "knocked out" some of the activity of the thyroid gland. This immune component might sit in waiting for your whole life, so on its own, it may not mean much. But if you have high TPO *and* you have a mild hypothyroid pattern, your health-care provider will likely consider medical treatment sooner than someone without any circulating TPO.

> ### Dr. Maurer on Thyroid Prescriptions:
>
> *Finding the thyroid hormone prescription that works best for you must be a collaborative effort between you and your health-care provider. But don't look for a prescription to miraculously provide you with the healthy metabolism you want. There are divisive opinions held about the kind of thyroid hormone that is prescribed to treat hypothyroidism: T4 alone, T4 with T3, natural glandular thyroid, customized ratios of T4 and T3, etc. A prescriber must be familiar with the various options, as well as which one is more appropriate for a particular individual. The prescription, regardless of whether a theory claims it is better or worse, only offers an incomplete solution. Part of the problem is that people are looking for the thyroid prescription to solve all of their metabolic symptoms. Hypothyroidism affects all of your tissues; it is not defined as merely the reduction in circulating hormone. And as I have mentioned in other places in this book,* it is common for people with a hypothyroid tendency to also have other metabolic thrifty behaviors like insulin resistance. *The food, fitness, and nutritional steps of The Blood Code are your way to complement any prescription for a thyroid-related condition.*

Your basal body temperature: If you have read this far into the thyroid chapter, you might have a question about why I have not acknowledged the basal body temperature (BBT) as a measurement of thyroid activity. Measured with an accurate thermometer first thing in the morning, the use of your BBT to identify hypothyroid activity is inadequate at best, and wildly misleading at worst. While thyroid hormones do influence metabolic function and temperature, they are the lesser among many other hormones and messenger molecules involved in thermoregulation.[14]

Thyroid hormones, like all other hormones in your body, interact with everything else. As your metabolism and overall fitness improves, the compounds in your body that regulate the activation and deactivation of T3 will improve as well. As you complete the steps in The Blood Code, your overall fitness and dietary needs, along with your energy, mood, and cellular metabolism, should all become more balanced.

Step Four: Adjust Your Blood Code Diet

Food is an important part of a balanced diet.
—Fran Lebowitz, stylish author

Key Dietary Concept: *We pay back our energy, we don't pay it forward.*

I will dare to use an economics reference here: The no-debt, cash economy does not work in your body. For anything meaningful to ever get done, there is always some debt/return that has to take place. Your body breaks itself down to get through the next few hours, to days, and then rebuilds itself within close to the same time frame. Your metabolism comprises two opposing yet complementary processes: anabolism and catabolism. *Anabolism* is the building of complex tissue; *catabolism* is the break-down process in which energy is released.

We are mistakenly given the message that what we eat is meant to provide for the next few hours of energy, or for some upcoming activity. In the evolution of our human body, we always had to do some activity on an empty stomach to *procure* the thing we were going to eat, and then we needed more time to prepare it before we could benefit from the calories. With this in mind, it should be no surprise that we are hormonally wired to use our tissue reserves for any activity and baseline energy. When you eat, your meal will be used to repair and replace what was broken down in the prior hours to days.

Are you ready for that? Eating *always* triggers an anabolic process. After a meal, hormones get secreted that tell your body to save the energy just ingested and rebuild what was broken down. Insulin is the chief anabolic hormone. This is a wildly empowering concept if you pause and think about it. Every day, every workout, every night, you break down a part of yourself. Your next meal provides the building blocks and the hormonal message to rebuild what you've lost. If you need to replace the sugars and fats that are stored in your body, dietary carbohydrates such as fruits and starches work great.

But, if you already wear enough adipose tissue, have enough circulating fats (as triglycerides), or have normal to high blood sugar, you had better reduce the foods that trigger and fund this storage process. If you have high blood sugar already, why eat a piece of fruit? You need to exercise on an empty stomach and allow your body to rightly use what it has stored; then, choose foods like vegetables with the right mix of nutrient-dense proteins and fats to provide your body with what it needs to rebuild itself, healthier than it was. *Again, every meal allows you the chance to rebuild in a smarter and healthier way.*

The Metabolic Effects of Carbs, Fats, and Proteins

As you may have already noticed in this book, the words *carbohydrate* and *carb* are used interchangeably. While it may not be a Scrabble word, *carb* is an accepted part of our lexicon in conversation and on food labels.

Carbs: Carbohydrates cause a strong release of insulin and trigger your body to store and save most of what you just ate. This process helps you prepare for the next period of no food, like overnight. Insulin is the primary hormone that signals you to store sugars and make and store fat; insulin also prevents the breakdown of fats you stored previously.

Proteins: Protein-rich foods also trigger insulin release, albeit to a lesser degree than carbs. Remember: Insulin has an anabolic action. Dietary protein signals the hormonal message to "store and rebuild." Proteins are the building blocks of all your tissues. Diets rich in protein have been shown to reduce food cravings and improve athletic recovery. Your body only burns protein for energy as a last resort, preferring fats instead (free fatty acids).

Fats: Dietary fats provide the preferred energy for your body. At rest, you burn more calories from fat than glucose. The irony here is that "fat burning" happens when you are at rest—*as long as insulin is not high!* Unlike carbs or proteins, dietary fats trigger no insulin release. Therefore, despite sounding contrary, high-fat/low-carb diets result in more overall fat loss, as fatty acids become a more-available fuel source. Dietary fats are proven to make you more satisfied and result in better self-regulation of daily caloric intake.

Appreciate the simplicity here: You have only three dietary materials to work with—carbs, fat, and protein. They are the only building blocks of your entire diet. Imagine if chemistry class were based upon a periodic table that listed only three elements; pretty easy, right? The confusion arises when one of the three is reduced.

In the early 1970s in the United States, dietary fat was suddenly named the villain. Low-fat foods inundated the marketplace, and from 1980 onward, Americans successfully reduced their total—and, especially, saturated—fat intake. Toward our collective ill health, carbohydrates catastrophically replaced those calories. If you want to read more on the historical reasons for the infamous low-fat diet and the consequences it brought, a particularly good book details our low-fat mistake: *Fat Land: How Americans Became the Fattest People in the World,* by Greg Critser.

Diet and nutrition in The Blood Code will be the easiest science class you have ever taken. There are only three foodstuffs to choose from. If one is decreased, the other two make up the difference. I, like you, perhaps, have the mild insulin-resistance trait. If I were to abide by the "low-fat" recommendations, I would quickly move toward type 2 diabetes. Why is a low-fat diet so bad for the 40 to 50 percent of people who, like me, carry the insulin-resistance trait?

Let's use the example of a popular food, like 8 ounces of yogurt, and see how the low-fat problem plays out:

Whole plain yogurt (8 oz.): 152 total calories, about *30 percent are carbs.*

8 grams fat	72 calories	47% are fat
9 grams protein	36 calories	24% are protein
11 grams carbs	**44 calories**	**29% are carbs**

Nonfat plain yogurt (8 oz.): only 112 calories, but the *carb content doubles to 60 percent.*

0 grams fat	0 calories	0% are fat
11 grams protein	44 calories	39% are protein
17 grams carbs	**68 calories**	**61% are carbs**

Nonfat yogurt has less taste and triggers less *satiety* (the satisfied feeling that helps you eat less in subsequent meals on that day). So, nonfat yogurt is usually sweetened with about 5 teaspoons of sugar.

A popular nonfat organic vanilla yogurt (8 oz.): 168 calories, a whopping *80 percent are carbs.*

0 grams fat	0 calories	0% are fat
9 grams protein	36 calories	21% are protein
33 grams carbs	**132 calories**	**79% are carbs**

You cannot effectively control insulin resistance and eat low-fat foods. Period. In fact, if you reduce your carbs, you will need to *add* dietary fat.

Let's turn the yogurt serving into something better: at 144 calories, *only 20 percent are carbs.*

Blood Code Diet serving: Whole plain yogurt, at a small volume of only *4 ounces*, with ten pecan halves (which are 90 percent fat and plenty of fiber) looks like this:

10 grams fat	90 calories	62% are fat
6 grams protein	24 calories	17% are protein
7.5 grams carbs	**30 calories**	**21% are carbs**

The dietary fat in this serving helps you feel satisfied. Studies show that you will naturally be satisfied with less total calories—with full-fat yogurt and the fat and fiber from nuts, you will be less likely to need a snack, and will eat less throughout the day. It's important to realize that the food-processing industry does *not* want you to do this. Their profits are dependent upon you eating more, not less. Your Blood Code Diet might be bad news for this industry, but it is liberating, good news for you.

If your goal is to cut calories, don't cut the fat out of the food. Leave the fats in and *eat less volume*. When dietary fats are a major part of your diet, you will be satisfied with fewer calories. But beware of processed foods: Studies have shown that this does not hold true if you choose processed foods with alluring "flavors, natural or artificial," because these compounds are designed, in part, to get you to eat *more* of the branded food.

A word about calories: As a matter of physical science, a calorie is absolute; however, nutritional experts are wrong to simplistically chant that "a calorie is a calorie." This adage ignores the different metabolic effects of foodstuffs on different people. Studies that compare weight-loss diets have repeatedly shown that low-carb/high-fat diets provide statistically greater weight loss than equal-caloric diets that are higher in carbohydrates.

> Every time you eat, your body sends hormonal signals to store and save what was eaten, and if you are one of those people who are really good at storing fat and sugar, high-carb foods will trigger you to store more.

The next step to fulfilling your healthful diet from your Blood Code is to "check" your carbohydrate intake. What is a simple carb? What is a complex carb? How much carb do you need, and how much is too much? Let's start with the carbohydrates.

Dietary Carbohydrates

I used to always equate carbs with energy, and that just doesn't seem to be the case.
—Patricia M., seventy-six, who eliminated type 2 diabetes with The Blood Code

You now know more about your personalized carbohydrate tolerance. As mentioned in the introduction, more Americans are likely to develop type 2 diabetes in their lifetime than have blue eyes. Insulin resistance is not a disease; it's not a genetic mistake that happened to help your ancestors to survive and reproduce while they ate few "storage carbohydrates" throughout the last ice age. Proteins and fats can total most of the calories you take in for a day. In nutrition-speak, there are essential amino acids and essential fats, but there are no "essential" carbohydrates, since you can make glucose readily from your body fats and, with more effort, from proteins. Therefore, choose the carbohydrate foods that deliver the most nutrient-dense punch, without putting you in storage mode. Vegetables, you will see, pack the most nutrients with the least carbohydrate load to your body.

Go ahead and fill in your carbohydrate goals per meal. The food lists that follow will allow you to add up the grams of carbs per meal. Your carbohydrate code is from Step Three: Putting It All Together (see page 87).

Fill in your carbohydrate code based upon your insulin resistance:

Breakfast: _____ grams

Lunch: _____ grams

Dinner: _____ grams

Your Carbohydrate Code:

Without insulin resistance or high insulin:
Breakfast: 30–40 grams
Lunch: 50–80 grams
Dinner: 50–80 grams

Slightly insulin-resistant or *slightly* high insulin:
Breakfast: 15–25 grams
Lunch: 40–60 grams
Dinner: 40–60 grams

Moderately insulin-resistant or *moderately* high insulin:
Breakfast: 10–20 grams
Lunch: 20–40 grams
Dinner: 20–40 grams

Severely insulin-resistant or *severely* high insulin:
Breakfast: 5–10 grams
Lunch: 10–15 grams
Dinner: 10–15 grams

A Word about the Glycemic Index and Why It Does Not Work!

The *glycemic index* is a popular way to numerically grade carbohydrate foods based upon the criteria of how much and how quickly the food results in elevated glucose in the bloodstream. This laboratory-derived list of foods is found in every reference work on diet and nutrition. The glycemic index is inappropriately but commonly used as evidence that a particular food is "good" or "bad." The logic of the glycemic index follows that good carbs are slow to result in glucose in the bloodstream, while bad carbs are faster to result in measurable blood glucose. Of course, foods that have no carbohydrate content are not on this scale, so fats and proteins have no inherent glycemic response.

There are problems with the overly simplistic glycemic index. Here are three reasons why you will not find the ubiquitous "glycemic index" in *The Blood Code:*

Reason #1: Food combination, like in a "balanced meal," is not accounted for in the glycemic index. *Fat and soluble fiber with the meal* effectively lowers the glycemic index of any carbohydrate food at that meal. The same effect is also seen if fermented foods and vinegar are added to a carbohydrate meal.

Reason #2: Excess glucose from carbs can clearly aggravate insulin resistance, but too much pure protein and large-volume meals trigger a problematic release of insulin, despite their lack of effect on blood sugar.[1]

Reason #3: I have saved the biggest reason for last: *Fructose!* Fructose is very low on the glycemic index, so it actually ends up in the "good" category, but fructose delays its harmful effect. Your body cannot immediately access the glucose molecule bound up in the fructose molecule. Many hours after you eat, fructose—whether from fruit or a processed sugar—gets converted into glucose, glycogen, lactate, and fat *in the liver.* There is a strong and adverse impact on the liver itself;

fatty liver and insulin resistance are made worse through the ingestion of fructose. It is swiftly turned into fatty liver, and can strongly trigger insulin resistance. The glycemic index of foods wrongly rewards high-fructose foods, because the index is only attentive to immediate glucose in the bloodstream; the delayed and harmful effect of fructose is neglected.[2]

Simple Sugars and Fructose: Why to Avoid Them

There are only three simple sugars: glucose, galactose, and fructose. *Glucose* is a simple, ready energy source for your cells. *Galactose* is one of the simple sugars behind the milk sugar, lactose. *Fructose* is found as free fructose in high-fructose corn syrup and honey, and it is found in its bound form in all table sugar, which is 50 percent fructose by weight. Free fructose just does not go bad; this is why honey can be left out, and why foods with enough high-fructose corn syrup can remain on a shelf for many years, with no visible adverse effects.

Why Fructose Is Worse, But Sugar Is Still Bad

The demonization of fructose in the last decade caused Big Agra industry pundits to call foul. They claim that their cheap, industrialized "high-fructose corn syrup," which is manufactured to contain either 42 percent or 55 percent fructose content, gets a bad rap, and they claim that evidence shows regular cane sugar is no better. Well, regular cane sugar is 50 percent fructose, so they are right; cane sugar is no better than high-fructose corn syrup. But they are also wrong; the fructose component may be the primary problem with excess sugar intake, feeding obesity, fatty liver, and insulin resistance.[3] *No person, with or without insulin resistance, should consume more than 20 grams of fructose per day.*

Sweetener type (per Tbsp)	Sugar (grams)	Fructose content (grams)
Agave	12	7–10
Honey	17	8.5
Maple syrup	14	7
Sugar/Cane sugar	12	6

Natural and processed sweeteners need to be counted carefully because of their concentrated fructose sugar, lack of nutrition, and fiber. Fruits are another potential source of fructose.

High–fructose fruits to avoid/limit*	Fructose (g)
2 medjool dates	15
1.5–oz. box of raisins	13
1 medium pear	11
1 medium apple	10
1 medium mango	8
3 dried figs	6
1 cup diced watermelon	5
1 banana	5
Misc. melons / 3 oz.	4
10 grapes	4
cherries/pineapple/papaya / 3 oz.	4
1 nectarine/apricot/plum	4
1 kiwi/guava	4
large blueberries/strawberries / 3 oz.	3
1 orange/grapefruit	3
lemons/limes/tomatoes	<3

If you have no insulin resistance, limit the high-fructose fruits, but if you express mild to severe insulin resistance, most fruit, especially those with fructose levels above 3g/serving, should be avoided.

Simple Sugar Summary

Simple sugar comes from sweeteners, fruit sugar, and milk sugar (lactose). Vegetables, legumes, and grains have no fructose, and have insignificant simple sugar content; they are referred to as *complex carbs.*

Complex Carbohydrates and The Blood Code Diet

A *complex carbohydrate* means that the glucose comes from a compound called *polysaccharide,* a molecule that remarkably resembles the stored form of sugar in mammals called glycogen. As mentioned above, vegetables, beans, and grains contain the complex carb, although there are a few exceptions (e.g., corn and beets, which are used to make processed sugar, but in their natural, whole-food state, have an inconsequential 2 to 4 percent simple sugar content).

With complex carbs, what you see is what you get. The carb content gets readily absorbed and is with you for the next several hours. There is no delayed blood sugar effect to your liver, as happens with fructose.

Many books and diet experts wrongly claim that complex carbs are good for people with insulin resistance. They go so far as to tell people with type 2 diabetes that they should switch from simple sugars to complex carbs. This is *not* a trade that cures. Certainly, you should choose complex carbs instead of simple carbs whenever possible, but for the sake of your Blood Code, a carb is a carb. Choose vegetable sources of starch, rather than juice or sugar. However, you can't switch from a candy bar with 40 grams of carb to a whole-wheat bagel with 40 grams of carb and think that by doing so, you will improve your prediabetes. There are ways to slow and offset the speed at which the carb hits your bloodstream.

Here is how to balance a carb into a meal.

Carbs in Balance

Carbohydrates in your Blood Code Diet need to be *part* of a meal, not the *whole* meal. Unopposed carbohydrates cause a greater sugar effect when eaten on their own compared to when they are part of a meal that can slow down the absorption.

Three food components can significantly lower the harmful sugar effect of a meal: dietary fats, fiber, and fermented foods.

Fats with a meal: If a meal contains a starchy carbohydrate like rice, with the addition of fatty broth or butter, the glucose from the carb will absorb more slowly, and you will have a healthier insulin response. Furthermore, studies show that people self-regulate to a lower food intake if adequate dietary fat is part of the meal. Foods like fattier proteins, olive oil, tree nuts, and avocados are good staples to add to your new dietary program.

Fermented foods offer countless benefits. Metabolically, the beneficial bacteria in cultured foods have "digested" part of the sugars for you. There is less lactose sugar in plain yogurt than the milk from which it was made. Fermented foods also alter the rate of sugar absorption; studies show that adding a cultured food—even a couple spoonfuls of sauerkraut—to a meal lowers the carb effect of the rest of the meal. Plain yogurt and cultured vegetables are a good place to start for your Blood Code Diet.

Soluble fiber is so named because it is soluble in water. The ability for a food to hold water tells of the soluble fiber content, and has the effect of creating a feeling of fullness without overeating calories. The soluble fibers also hold on to sugars from the food and release them at a slower rate, allowing a healthier insulin response. Both soluble and insoluble fibers are carbohydrates, but large cellulose fibers do not get absorbed in your digestive tract, so they "don't count." This gives rise to the term *net carbs*.

Natural net carbohydrates: Carbohydrate foods have varying amounts of fiber. Legumes tend be regarded as a high-fiber food, but even though beans are rich in soluble fiber, to get 8 grams of fiber, you need to ingest 24 grams of total carb. On the other hand, an avocado delivers a whopping 9 grams of fiber in only 11 total grams of total carb, so the "net carb" from an avocado is only 2 grams.

The term *net carb* has been abused by the processed-food industry; they mix and blend difficult-to-digest fibers into things like pasta and bread, and then subsequently claim that they have made bread products that are "low net carb." Apart from the bloating and digestive upset that often results from these foods, they also frequently cause higher blood sugar than expected, based on the label claims. Do *not* rely on processed foods that claim low net carbs. Nature provides soluble fiber in traditional whole foods; therefore, I'll use the designation *natural net carbs* throughout this section.

Choose the Carbohydrates in Your Blood Code Diet

Staple Carbohydrates: Four to Six Servings per Day

The following are the carbohydrate foods that should be staples in your diet. In short, vegetables and more vegetables. With their high soluble fiber and low-carb content, they help to maintain your healthiest blood sugar levels. Many of these foods have been part of the human diet for millennia, so it's no surprise that your immune system has an affinity for these nutrient-laden gems.

Studies repeatedly show that those who eat the most vegetables win over those who eat the least, whether the end point is weight, diabetes, cancer, or heart disease. Vegetables contain numerous vitamins and minerals, and compounds that have impressive and unique health benefits—albeit, with chemical-sounding names like lutein, flavonoids, and zeaxanthin. Don't get caught up with all the different compound names; just realize that these important phytonutrients come from plants, and there are no substitutes.

Dark greens: I often see posters in my local schools stating that we should eat colorful fruits and vegetables, but the poster neglects the basics of chemistry: Dark green trumps, and contains, all colors. We are able to enjoy the lovely colors of our New England autumn foliage when the green color recedes from the leaves, allowing us to see the orange, red, and yellow shades that were there all along. Dark, leafy greens contain all the benefits of colorful fruits and vegetables, and then some.

Hearty dark greens like kale, chard, collards, beet and turnip greens, leeks, okra, and spinach all need to be cooked. Each of these vegetables (except the kale) contains an irritating and nutrient-binding compound called *oxalic acid*. Too much oxalic acid can result in kidney stones. Oxalic acid prevents the absorption of calcium, so even though these vegetables have a significant iron and calcium content, the minerals are not bioavailable to humans in the raw form. Cooking these vegetables does free up some of the calcium and iron as the cell walls break down. Chefs and farmers will also use the trick of freezing the vegetables so the expansion of water breaks the cell walls. This provides healthier absorption of the key minerals, although it only reduces the oxalic acid content by a small amount. Those prone to kidney stones should develop a fondness for kale, which contains no oxalic acid.

Root vegetables: Potatoes, sweet potatoes, carrots, parsnips, and turnips all provide carbohydrate with fiber, and minimal to no protein and fat. Potato and sweet potato provide more carbs per pound than many of the other roots.

The substantial carb content of root vegetables needs to be counted, and eaten, in accordance with your Blood Code. As you reduce the quantity of these starchy foods, you will need to increase dietary fats; luckily, these vegetables make good vehicles for traditional fats. Boil up and mash parsnips and carrots, but add plenty of butter and cultured cream, and the carb content will be less than 20 percent due to the addition of dietary fats.

The Blood Code Diet Staple Carbohydrates

Per 3-ounce serving, these veggies have less than 5 grams (usually less than 3 grams) of carbs. Three ounces by weight is a medium carrot, a small bowlful of broccoli, or a large bowl of mushrooms.

Vegetables are a good place to use traditional fats—coconut oil, olive oil, butter, or other quality animal fats like duck, chicken, or lard

Blood Code Staple Carbohydrates
One at breakfast / one to two at lunch and dinner:

Artichoke, whole and hearts
Asparagus
Avocado
Beans, string and green
Bok choy
Broccoli
Brussels sprouts
Cabbage (also as coleslaw, sauerkraut, kimchi)
Carrots
Cauliflower
Celery
Cucumber
Eggplant
Fennel root
Greens (collard, beet, turnip, kale, Swiss chard, leeks)
Herbal greens (parsley, cilantro, etc.)
Lettuces, all varieties
Mushrooms, any variety
Okra
Onions/shallots/garlic
Peppers, all colors
Radishes
Snow peas, snap peas in the pod
Spaghetti squash
Spinach (steamed, creamed, wilted, sautéed)
Sprouts from alfalfa or beans
Tomato/tomatillo/salsas
Turnip/parsnip/rutabaga
Yellow/zucchini squash

The Blood Code Diet: Starchy Vegetables

Starchy vegetables are a concentrated source of carbohydrate energy, so just stay within your individual Blood Code allowance. Compared to grains, root vegetables and winter squash are higher in nutrients and easier to digest (3 ounces is about 100 grams).

Starchy Vegetables:

Choose near the top	Amount	Natural Net Carb Content
Turnip	3 oz.	3 grams
Beet	3 oz.	4 grams
Carrot	3 oz.	5 grams
Winter squash / rutabaga	3 oz.	6 grams
*Corn	1 ear	12 grams
*Peas	3 oz.	14 grams
*Sweet potatoes	1 medium	20 grams
*White potatoes	1 medium	32 grams

* Note how these are substantially higher in carbs than the other root vegetables. Therefore, if you have moderate or severe insulin resistance, you should use the vegetables that are lower on the list (see the roasted root veggies in the meal planner, on page 225).

The Blood Code Diet: Beans/Legumes

Frequently mistaken as a high-protein food, bean dishes are less than 20 percent protein, and are best viewed as a fibrous starchy carbohydrate. The skin on a bean is wildly indigestible; long soaking processes are required to make legumes less irritating to your digestion. Traditionally the rinsed beans would be mixed with water, aromatic herbs, and salt, and placed in a hot place overnight. The following day, the beans are heated to evaporate some of the water. Beans have plenty of soluble fiber, but remain very difficult for most people to digest. Grains and beans have similar carbohydrate content.

Cooked Legumes (per 4 Tbsp, or 1/4 cup serving)*	Natural Net Carb Content
Lentils	6 grams
Garbanzo beans (chickpeas)	8 grams
Black beans / Navy Beans	9 grams
Adzuki beans	10 grams

Notice that the serving size is a paltry 4 level tablespoons of cooked beans.

A word about soybeans and peanuts, and why they should be avoided in their processed forms: These two legumes have been among the most processed and misused foods in the convenience-food culture. Soy products are apparently on shaky ground, as they have been associated with thyroid and other hormonal conditions.[4] Yet, on the other side, I've read other industry research that refers to soy products as some kind of miraculous *medical food*. (Somebody please tell me why this term makes soy—or any food, for that matter—more desirable?)

Soy protein isolate and *textured vegetable protein* are foods that did not exist in the human diet until a generation ago. The resultant processed foodstuff challenges your human digestive system. Over the past few thousand years that beans have been part of the human diet, soybeans were boiled, not extracted out to be soy flour and soy protein. I suspect the growing incidence of soy protein allergy is a result of our inability to digest the food in its processed form.

Peanuts went through a similar process. Peanuts were always boiled in various native cuisines. Boiled for an hour in salt water, fresh in their pods, the peanuts were eaten like the popular Japanese dish, edamame.

Only in the 1930s did the Skippy Corporation patent and begin the process of roasting the peanuts rather than boiling them, to make peanut butter. This caused an emulsification of the fats that allowed the product to be more spreadable. Just add sugar from jelly and you have the modern way peanuts are eaten. While spreadability meets the needs of convenience, nutrition and digestibility are radically compromised, challenging the human digestive and immune systems. Like soybeans and other legumes, skipping the process of boiling the peanut leaves the indigestible outer skin on the legume intact, causing stomach and digestive problems, poor nutrition, and potential allergies.

Grains and Breads: The Whole-Grain Myth Decoded

Many people get fixated on the color or "wholeness" of a grain. The only difference between whole-grain brown rice and white rice is the 1.5 grams of insoluble fiber that remains in the half-cup of cooked brown rice. The soluble fiber content is the same; this is why you use the same proportion of water to rice whether you're using brown or white. Other grains are the same; white flour and wheat flour differ only in the content of the indigestible grain husk.

Common myth states that the nutrients all get stripped away when the husk is removed, but the insoluble husk contains few absorbable nutrients. The insoluble husk also provides minimal to no difference in the glycemic effect. So if you prefer white rice, no worries; if you want more nutrients, cook the rice in vegetable or bone broth rather than water. Butter the finished product and eat less. A switch from white flour to whole-wheat flour will not improve your metabolism. Period.

Besides the indigestible fibers in whole-grain foods, gluten is another component of grain that may be difficult for you to digest. I have therefore separated the grains into non-gluten and gluten categories. In my clinical practice, I repeatedly see insulin resistance lurking behind the gluten-intolerance symptoms that many people experience, such as severe fatigue after meals. If you have high insulin, you will probably feel worse with bread, whether it contains gluten or not. Therefore, count the total carbs and only eat what you can tolerate.

The Blood Code Diet Grain Choices

Note the small quantity: *The serving size for the grains below is a meager 4 level tablespoons of cooked/prepared grain.* If you are moderately to severely insulin-resistant, you should avoid grains altogether; otherwise, you will regularly land above your carbohydrate range.

Easy-to-digest, "non-gluten" grains:

Grain	Natural net carb per 1/4 cup (note: this is only 4 Tbsp)
Oatmeal	6–7 grams
Rice, wild	7–8 grams
Corn grits	7–8 grams
Quinoa	9–10 grams
Rice	10–11 grams
Millet	10–11 grams
Crackers	Check labels

Hard-to-digest gluten grains:

Grain	Natural net carb per 1/4 cup (4 Tbsp)
Bulgur	6–7 grams
Couscous	9 grams
Pasta	9–11 grams
*Bread, any flour	15–25 grams/slice
Crackers	Check labels

Traditional sourdough breads are soaked in an acidic fermenting starter. This soaking process makes the bread a little easier to digest, and removes up to 20 percent of the carbohydrate from the bread. While this is an improvement, and a better bread choice, 20 grams to 17 grams still means that sourdough bread is a high-carb food. Bread products also have different density, and, therefore, different carbohydrate levels. A baguette in France, in my experience, is only 2 inches in diameter and weighs about as much as a few pencils; this airy bread product therefore has less carbs per piece than a dense, American-style baguette. You will have to choose accordingly.

AVOID THESE GRAINS

The following list includes grains that are extremely dense and difficult to digest. Granola is essentially raw, whole grain; experiencing gas and bloating six to eight hours after eating is remarkably common with this food. The industry effectively sells these processed-grain foods because the end result is formed into cool, patented shapes, and they maintain their crunch. The consumer should avoid them because of the excessively high-carb concentration and indigestibility.

Grain products	Total carbs
Bagels	50–70 grams
Boxed cereals	25–40 grams
Pizza dough	30–40 grams/slice
Granola	35–45 grams / half-cup serving
Granola bars	25–35 grams/bar

What Would a Bread-Free Diet Look Like?

What was there before sliced bread?
—Steven Wright, comedian

A word about "paleo" diets:

While I do think that we humans have adapted to dietary changes since the Stone Age, I appreciate many of the dietary and fitness ideas that come to people from the popularized "paleolithic diet." This diet has given people permission to live without grains, and therefore, obviously, without bread. This diet goes a step further and discourages the intake of dairy, beans, and many fruits. Most people pick up the paleolithic diet as a way of eating to feel better, and oftentimes it works great. But in my practice I have also seen people with low insulin that should not be on such a low-carb diet. If your Blood Code implies that you need to significantly reduce carbohydrates, the dietary ideas and principles of the paleolithic diets will parallel most of your dietary and fitness needs.

Dr. Maurer's Don'ts:

Two non-caloric and non-carb ways to worsen your insulin resistance: *high-volume foods and artificial sweeteners.*

Large Meal Size

> *Never order food in excess of your body weight.*
> —Erma Bombeck

Stretching the stomach triggers a release of excess insulin, due to the gastric release of the hormones called incretins. Evolutionarily, an excessively high-volume meal was probably very high calorically, but the volume of the meal seems to be a separate trigger. There are outdated but popular weight-loss programs that promote high-volume, low-calorie foods; the misguided theory is to allow people to eat an excessive volume, knowing that since the food is empty, it counts less.

> **Stomach stretch example:** Three roasted chicken wings add up to about 240 calories, filling the volume of a lemon. Popcorn at the same caloric intake fills the volume of a football, at about 9 cups. Anatomically, your stomach is well designed to stretch; average post-meal distention is about 2 cups in size, the size of two large lemons. Greater than this, and the stretch receptors in your digestive tract signal a bigger release of insulin. It makes sense, right? If the mother lode of food volume just entered, you'd better get ready to store, store, store.

Your goal, then, is to eat smaller-volume, more-nutrient-rich and calorically dense foods. Dietary fats allow you to do this. I know that you're smart enough to see the difference between a $20 bill and a $5 bill; the $20 bill contains more value in the same size piece of paper.

In the case of food density, 1 Tbsp of oatmeal has 8 calories; 1 Tbsp of chicken has about 30 calories; and 1 Tbsp of butter has 90 calories. If I were to get my daily 3,000 calories from a grain-based diet, I would need to eat a volume of food larger than a soccer ball, and I would subsequently express my type 2 diabetes trait. In your Blood Code Diet, choose the more calorically dense foods: fats and dense proteins, with lower-volume cooked vegetables. The Blood Code Diet naturally leads you toward these calorically dense foods. I know that you will actually feel better and self-regulate more naturally toward a lifetime of dietary habits that will work best for you.[5]

Artificial Sweeteners

You can fool most of the people some of the time, but you can't fool us anymore.

For many years, epidemiological data have demonstrated an association between artificial sweetener use and weight gain, but cause and effect is not always crystal clear. Animal studies show that artificial sweeteners play an active metabolic role that contributes to insulin resistance. In human studies, people who ingest more artificial sweeteners have more weight gain. Is it due to extra eating elsewhere in the day? Is it due to some insulin-resistance trigger? Is there some other chemical effect that is unforeseen? Your body is wired to anticipate glucose entering the bloodstream, and at least for the past thousand generations, this went along with taste receptors detecting sweetness.

Given that it took the scientific community decades to prove that smoking might be harmful, it comes as no surprise that there is industry-led resistance to the claim that artificial sweeteners are a problem. These metabolically controversial, processed-food chemicals should be used very sparingly, or not at all.[6]

Dietary carbs in my diet . . .

I eat less carbs than others in my family. Breakfast includes eggs for the protein and fat, while the carb content is a low-carb veggie (chard, spinach, or kale), and while exercising regularly, a few fingerling potatoes or a couple of crackers or a half piece of toast. At lunch, if not leftovers, I will find picnic-style foods: some crackers, pickled veggies, a wedge of cheese, some cole-slaw (already made in the fridge); each food delivers some carb content. Dinner is a salad, a sautéed green, some roasted or grilled veggies, and then a protein. Again, as my activity level increases, potatoes* offer a useful addition to my diet.

But I am human, and I regularly see the damaging emotional effects that come from food neuroses, as people struggle to be perfect. As a result, I am not overly controlling with my carb restriction. If my blood tests continue to look good with my current habits, I know that even though I'm imperfect, I'm good enough.

—Dr. Richard Maurer

* *Pasta, white rice, or a baguette will all be used here, in limited quantities.*

Dietary Fats

If you have been limiting them, you must reintroduce dietary fats:
You need to accept fat as an inherently important component of your diet and cuisine. Dietary fats, and especially the saturated fats, need to be put *back* into your healthful dietary discourse.

A farmer knows that there is a limit to how much protein an acre of land can sustainably produce. Dietary fats provide essential calories that fill in the protein and vegetable landscape of your diet; for example, the skin on the chicken is as worthy a calorie as the lean meat, and must remain part of the meal.

A chef knows that good cuisine requires good fats. Not the processed trans fats of the margarine years, but real, traditional fats that have been part of human evolution and cuisine for millennia. A local Maine chef is acclaimed in part because of the miraculous flavor he gets out of potatoes through the addition of duck fat. It is such a lovely thing to cook with, and is the inspiration for his restaurant's name.

You must know that dietary fats will keep you in your metabolic sweet spot: There is no way you will effectively recover your metabolic health without fats as an integral part of your diet. Carbohydrate foods, especially simple sugars, trigger insulin release and storage. Protein foods also trigger insulin release and storage. All you have left is fats. If you eat half a stick of butter and chug a jigger of olive oil (not advisable, by the way), your body does not trigger an insulin response despite the 1,000 calories ingested. Olive oil receives accolades about its great health benefits, but the reason olive oil is so great is because it is an unprocessed, calorie-rich addition that is *not bad.* If you already have a problem with excess storage, eating excessive carb and protein foods that stimulate *more* storage will make your problem worse. You need plenty of neutral and healthful dietary fats along with your tolerable amount of the staple carbohydrates in order to nourish you without excess metabolic storage.

Dietary fats were not always seen as the villain: In 1841 the French Academy of Sciences published a treatise entitled "Obesity and Excessive Corpulence: The Various Causes and the Rational Means of Cure," by Dr. Jean-François Dancel. At this time science acknowledged that most mammals could be "fattened up by eating a diet rich in farinaceous products"—corn, rice, sorghum, etc. (Note: This is the feed-lot strategy still employed today to produce not the healthiest cattle, but certainly big and fatty cattle.)

In 1882 a German physician named Wilhelm Ebstein published a concise report entitled "Obesity and its Treatment." He argued that fatty foods were critical, as they induced a feeling of satiety. Therefore, his recommendations sounded something like this: "No sugar, potatoes, sweets, and only limited bread—while enjoying meat of every kind, especially fatty meats." Although he did offer one radical caveat . . . Ready for this? "Avoid eating too much food."

Reducing overall food intake, with starches and sweets specifically, remained the medical model for successful weight control for many generations. In 1940 another report, this time written by Dr. Hugo Rony of Northwestern University School of Medicine in Illinois, concluded that most people have a marked preference for sugary and/or starchy foods. This was based on responses Dr. Rony had gathered from interviews with a series of obese patients, when more than 80 percent of respondents indicated that these were the types of food they most desired.

Suddenly, over the past fifty years, headlines have mistakenly identified dietary fat as the fall guy. Investigative journalists have been hard at work, looking at both sides of the fat feud. Their work is invaluable for anyone looking for more insight into the fallacy of the "fat-is-bad" theory. The list of books and articles that vindicate dietary fats includes Michael Pollan's 2006 article, "Eating," in the *New York Times Magazine;* Barry Glassner's *The Gospel of Food: Everything You Think You Know about Food Is Wrong;* Gary Taubes's book, *Good Calories, Bad Calories: Challenging the Conventional Wisdom on Diet, Weight Control, and Disease; Fat Land:*

How Americans Became the Fattest People in the World, by Greg Critser; and *Real Food: What to Eat and Why,* by Nina Planck.

Saturated fat in your diet is desirable: As of 2013, researchers have finally caught up with the investigative journalists who found no evidence that dietary saturated fat was the actual root of heart disease risk. Research teams are more skilled at accounting and controlling for processed-food intake, including the Framingham Heart Study and the Nurses' Health Study, whose data displays no link between saturated fat and heart disease. If you're wondering why you have so often heard the erroneous claim "Saturated fat is bad," the author of the 2013 study, Dr. Lawrence, is wondering too. He states, "[It] makes one wonder how saturated fats got such a bad reputation in the health literature."[7]

Yeah, it makes me wonder too. I have seen people with heart disease risk get worse by going on their doctor-recommended "low-fat diet." I have seen people with anxiety and panic attacks caused by the blood sugar instability that results from a low-fat diet. Conversely, I have seen children reduce their symptoms of autism after going from a low-fat diet to a diet rich in traditional, unprocessed dietary fats. If I, myself, were to eat the amount of food I require in a day as a low-fat diet, I would be type 2 diabetic within just a few years. Since there is no standing evidence to support the positive health effects of a low-fat diet, like Dr. Lawrence, it makes me wonder.

Fats in your Blood Code Diet are essential, both for building a healthy body and allowing your metabolism to run without the brakes being applied. Insulin is the metabolic brake in your body; it engages when you eat volume carbohydrate foods, like bread. You stop burning fat and start storing it. Dietary fat is nutrient-dense, which means that the calories come in a small volume. Dietary fats as they enter the bloodstream do not require or stimulate your insulin. Dietary fats, including saturated and monounsaturated fats alike, offer an efficient and long-burning package of calories that provides satiety and sustainable energy without contributing to extra insulin release. Dietary fats are the calories that keep you insulin-sensitive, with optimal energy throughout the day.

If Saturated Fat is Okay, What Are the Bad Fats?

#1 Hydrogenated oils: These include hydrogenated and partially hydrogenated oils. This process creates a great deal of the inarguably damaging "trans" fats.

#2 "No-fat" and "low-fat" products: These products are marketed based upon their fat content, or lack thereof; they have either more sugar or more chemicals to mimic the taste and/or texture of fat. To get the mouth feel of mayonnaise in a "low-fat" product is a miracle of the food chemical industry. The chemical end product may be good for them, but it's not good for you.

#3 Heated, whipped, or stored vegetable oils: Heating or cooking an oil promotes that oil to become oxidized, otherwise known as rancid. Rancid oil is unhealthful. Period. So when you cook, heat-stable oil must be used.

High-temperature cooking should be done with a saturated fat (e.g., coconut oil, butter/ghee, rendered animal fats such as chicken fat, lard, or duck fat).

Low-temperature (<350 degrees) cooking could be done with olive oil or sesame oil.

Cooking should not be done in the unstable polyunsaturated oils (PUFA) such as canola, corn, sunflower, safflower, flax, and soy oils. Commercial and industrial kitchens use these oils because they are cheap. Yes, these vegetable oils when heated are harmful to your health.

If you are looking for crackers, look for those that use olive oil or butter as the cooking oil, or those that use no oils, like traditional Scandinavian crackers. Nearly all commercial chips are cooked at high temperature in unstable PUFA oil and should be avoided.

#4 Too much omega-6 fat can be . . . too much: Nuts and seeds and vegetable oils (oils of corn, safflower, sunflower, sesame, soybean) contain high amounts of omega-6 fatty acids. Omega-3 fats, the essential fats that make cold-water fish such a health-promoting food, need to be in balance with the omega-6. The excessive commercial use of the cheap omega-6 PUFA oils has thrown this balance off. While omega-6 fats are technically essential (in small doses) for your health, too much leaves you prone to inflammation throughout your body.

Therefore, a daily adequate amount of nuts is about ten to fifteen almonds, or equivalent weight in other nuts.

How Much Dietary Fat Do You Need?

You have calculated your carbohydrate code for each meal, and there are only two foodstuffs left: protein and fats. Proteins are not a preferred "fuel" source, although proteins do help support your exceptionally important lean body strength, and will need to be increased. Fats are your preferred fuel/energy source; they provide energy that does not stress or contribute to insulin resistance. You will count your carbohydrate intake to ensure that you stay within your Blood Code. Fats do not need to be counted; dietary fats effectively trigger satiety, and you will likely appreciate the feeling of satisfaction that comes from a properly balanced, fats-rich meal.

A Case of Switching to Fats
Jennifer A., fifty-two years old

Jen was fifty-two years old when she came to see me, worried about her blood sugars. Two grandparents had diabetes later in life, and she wanted a different future. She never had a "weight problem," but had prediabetes on her 2011 test. She was afraid to give up the "low fat diet" her doctor had recommended, but saw the blood sugars rising and knew what *that* future looked like. She set her carb ranges for moderate insulin resistance (see page 108).

Test Date	12/5/11 Jen's low–fat diet	3/10/12 Blood Code diet
Triglyceride	102 mg/dL	68 mg/dL
HDL	48 mg/dL	60 mg/dL
TG:HDL ratio	2.1	1.1
HgbA1C	6.0 %	5.4 %
Fasting glucose	104 mg/dL	86 mg/dL
Fasting insulin	8 uIU/mL	6 uIU/mL
HOMA–IR	2.1	1.3

Jen continues to be surprised. "I thought I was eating pretty healthy before, but now, I feel better, my mood and energy are more even, and I feel more satisfied eating this way."

Dr. Maurer notes, "The shift from carbs to fats made the difference. Jen only moderately increased her protein intake: an extra egg, more chicken. Whereas her dietary fat intake went from 23 percent of calories to now close to 60 percent of her daily caloric intake."

Jen's Diet	Prior Low-Fat Diet Natural Net Carb in (##)	After Her Blood Code Diet Natural Net Carb in (##)
Breakfast	2 toast (36), one with 1/2 Tbsp butter, one with 1 Tbsp jam (11), banana (23) 70 grams of carb 300 total calories **Carbs = 70%** **17% from fat** (butter)	2 eggs, sautéed spinach and mushrooms in 1 Tbsp butter, 1/2 grapefruit (10) 10 grams of carb 300 total calories **Carbs = 13%** **66% from fat** (eggs and more butter)
Lunch	Chicken salad wrap (50 from wrap), small bag of an organic crunchy thing (24), apple (21), water 95 grams of carb 700 total calories **Carbs = 54%** **29% from fats** (mayo and chips)	Twice the chicken salad (5), a bed of greens (1) w/1 Tbsp of olive oil, about 10 croutons (14), avocado from home (3) 23 grams of carb 700 total calories **Carbs = 13%** **70% from fats** (mayo, avocado, olive oil, and croutons)
Dinner	1 cup cooked rice (44), 1/2 cooked beans (20), 2 soft tacos (26), baked fish, lettuce, salsa (5), 2 oz. cheese (1), beer (12) 108 grams of carb 900 total calories **Carbs = 48%** **22% from fat** (cheese)	No rice, 1/2 cup beans (20), twice the fish (0), lettuce w/olive oil, salsa (5), 2 oz. cheese (1), 3 Tbsp cultured cream (2), one glass wine (4) 32 grams of carb 900 total calories **Carbs = 14%** **50% from fat** (cheese, cream, olive oil)

Sources of the Different Dietary Fats:

- **Omega-3 fats:** Fatty fish and fish oils, egg yolks, some seeds
- **Omega-6 fats:** Most nuts and seeds, especially pumpkin/sun-flower/sesame/flax seeds, almonds, pecans, walnuts, brazil nuts; all seeds, nuts, and nut butters must be *raw*—not roasted
- **Omega-9 fats:** Artichoke hearts, avocados, olives, and olive oil
- * **Short-chain fats:** Butter—try to find organic, local, or "cultured" butter
- * **Medium-chain fats:** Coconut oil
- * **Longer-chain fats:** Predominantly from animal/meat sources, these fats supply a mix of omega-6 and omega-3 essential fats, along with saturated fats; grass-fed beef and lamb have been shown to contain an especially healthy fatty acid profile.

Omega-3, -6, and -9 fats are the beneficial nutrients that are used to build healthy tissues throughout your body; omega-3 and -6 are "essential" fats.

* These are dietary saturated fats, which are stable with heat and cooking methods, and provide metabolically desirable sources of energy.

Nuts and Seeds in The Blood Code Diet

Nuts do provide an effective way to add fats and some fiber to many foods (e.g., chicken with cashews; yogurt with pecans; and salads with slivered almonds). Since most of you will use nutritious and fibrous nuts in your diet, let's clarify some rules:

First, a peanut is not a nut. You can read more about peanuts and soybeans in the legume section of the carbohydrate chapter (see page 119—120). In your Blood Code Diet, roasted peanuts and peanut butter are *not* healthful staple foods.

Second, tree nuts are *not* high-protein foods. The protein content is negligible—only about 10 percent. Therefore, they are to be used as condiments with other foods, not as a main course. For example: Fourteen raw almonds contain 100 calories: 85 percent fat, 13 percent protein, 2 percent carb. Ten pecan halves contain 104 calories: 92 percent fat, 4 percent protein, 4 percent carb. Seeds similarly contain 80 percent fats and no more than 10 percent protein.

Third, nuts that are roasted at a high temperature are rancid. While most tree nuts taste "nuttier" when roasted at a high temperature, the delicate omega-6 fatty acid will quickly oxidize, or go rancid. The subsequent free-radical-rich rancid oil promotes inflammation in your body. Commercial roasting of nuts is done at a high temperature, and anything greater than about 160 to 180 degrees Fahrenheit will result in oxidation of the nut oils. Therefore, buy raw nuts, not roasted.

Fourth, too many nuts are difficult to digest. Some people have a great deal of trouble digesting fiber-rich nuts. This might be due to excess intake. Your solution? Eat less. But another reason might be the indigestible compounds in the skin of the nuts, which protects the nut from being digested by bugs and animals while it grows on the tree. When dry, the nut is still protected, but once soaked in water, the irritating compound breaks down; this is to prepare the nut for germination after a nice, wet location is present for the nut or seed. You can mimic this process to improve the digestibility.

Soaking nuts and seeds, especially nuts that have the skin on them, will do this. You can follow the steps below for almonds, pecans, walnuts, and pumpkin seeds:

1) Rinse the nuts in a mesh colander.
2) Cover with water and soak at room temperature overnight, or for at least four hours.
3) Place in a thin layer on a pan* in an oven at low temperature, essentially as low as the oven will go. Less than 150 degrees is best. Drying might take eight hours or more.
4) Let cool and store just like any dried nut.

* For flavor: Add salt or other spices prior to drying if desired.

Staple Dietary Fats for Your Kitchen

Olive oil: You should never buy premade salad dressing; all store-bought dressings contain inferior oils, and, usually, unwanted sweeteners. Make your own dressing with good extra virgin olive oil as the base.

Mayonnaise should have real egg yolks and quality oil, and again, is something that's very easy to make yourself. I recommend using fresh-made commercial oils, like the Delouis fils brand. (Note: Fresh-made mayo has a shorter shelf life.)

Crème fraîche is a traditional cultured cream; it is essentially like yogurt, made out of cream rather than milk.

Great cooking oils for high-temperature cooking include coconut oil, clarified butter, and quality rendered animal fats such as chicken fat, duck fat, or lard. *Great cooking oils for lower-temperature cooking,* or to add to food that is already cooked, include olive oil, butter, and cold-pressed sesame oil.

Dietary fat staples in my diet . . .

My family of five goes through a liter of olive oil and one to two pounds of butter per week. We use crème fraîche and organic mayonnaise regularly, and they are always in the fridge. I splurge and buy duck fat to sauté or roast vegetables. Raw slivered almonds, pecans, and sunflower seeds are regular additions to salads and whole plain yogurt. All cuts of meat are full fat, skin on, etc.

Dietary Proteins

How much protein do you need?

You need 0.5 to 1.0 gram per pound of lean body mass (LBM). (For metric, this is 1.1 to 2.2 grams of protein per kg of lean body weight.) LBM is your total body weight minus your percentage of body fat. This number comes from your skin-fold calipers. Strenuous exercise and exertion will increase your body's demand for muscle and tissue repair, and, subsequently, dietary protein needs will be on the higher side of the range.

Protein Needs Based on Lean Body Mass

Weight (lbs.)	Body fat %	Lean body mass (lbs.)	Your Protein Requirement
125	15%	105	50–100 grams
	20%	100	
	25%	94	
150	15%	128	60–120 grams
	20%	120	
	25%	114	
200	15%	170	75–160 grams
	20%	160	
	25%	150	

What about too little protein?

While your body *can* survive on less protein, recovery will be compromised, such as recovery from an illness, or recovery from an injury or activity. Perhaps you can live successfully on less protein than .5 grams/

pound of LBM if you are older, celibate, passive, and with no underlying health problem.

What about too much protein?

Rarely does anyone's diet need to exceed 200 grams of protein per day. If you are not exercising significantly, you will likely settle at 60 to 100 grams of protein. If you have a regular practice of intense exercise or high-resistance exercise, you will require 100 to 200 grams of protein. No organization has come up with a hard-and-fast rule about the optimal amount of dietary protein for an individual. Research has shown that high-protein diets are likely safe for the vast majority of people. And even for athletes, the timing of a meal, the mix of specific amino acids, and the athlete's unique metabolic response to the meal play as much of a role as the total amount of protein ingested daily.[8]

What protein amount is "just right" for you?

When you restrict dietary carbohydrates in your Blood Code Diet, you will be eating more from dietary proteins and fats. To review, your body produces the hormone insulin primarily in response to carbohydrate intake, but you also release some insulin—about one-third less insulin than carbs—in response to dietary protein.[9] Research has confirmed that ample dietary protein in a carbohydrate-restrictive diet improves the maintenance of lean body mass during weight loss, the control of blood sugars, and self-regulated appetite control. [10] Adequate protein at breakfast is especially important for weight loss, blood sugar control, mood, and concentration.

If you are insulin-resistant and physically active, protein in the meal following a strenuous workout will release plenty of insulin, and will support your muscle mass. But if you add a bunch of carbs to your protein, like rice with boneless/skinless chicken, you will have way too much insulin release. This is probably why traditional cultures prepared proteins and carbs with plenty of fat.

Whole Foods in The Blood Code Diet

Whole food means that all the natural nutrients are present. When you choose chicken, the bone is in and the skin is on.

Boneless, skinless chicken is the white bread of the protein world. When you choose an egg, eat the white *and* the yolk. Choose beef with a natural fat content (no cut of beef is more than 85 percent lean, so avoid those products that claim over 90 percent lean), and cook it with the bone in whenever possible. The micronutrients, vitamins, and minerals in meats and fish are mostly found in the bones, organs, and the meat "juices" that come from slow cooking.

Take the extra steps toward food quality. As you eat higher on the food chain, pay closer attention to quality and farming impact. Make an effort to purchase your protein foods from sources that are organic, grass-fed, local, or at least "natural." For fish sources, the Monterey Bay Aquarium offers a website and app to help you locate and choose regional and sustainable fish and shellfish.

Protein Content and Dietary Sources

MEATS AND POULTRY:
Contain 25 to 30 grams of protein per 3 raw ounces (not including bones)
Chicken/turkey: bone in and skin on
Wild-game meats
Grass-fed beef or lamb

Organic/natural organ meats can be prepared into pate and terrine and spreads. Virtually all traditional cuisines have a favorite food containing organ meats (e.g., scrapple, cretons, blood sausage, liverwurst, etc.).

FISH:
Contain 20 to 25 grams of protein per 3 ounces
Look for sustainable fish in your area. In the northern areas of the United States, we look for anchovies, bluefish, catfish, cod, clams, crab meat, haddock, halibut, herring, lobster, mackerel, mussels, oysters, salmon, sardines, scallops, and shrimp.

Avoid those fish with the highest mercury content; these are the big predator fish, like swordfish, shark, and large tuna. The fish with the lowest mercury content are small fish, like pollock, sardines, herring, etc.

Try whole sardines (25 grams of protein per can), canned salmon, and anchovies; these all have bones in, and therefore provide high levels of calcium, iron, and other nutrients.

EGGS:
Contain 6 to 8 grams of protein per large chicken egg

DAIRY:
Plain milk and yogurt have 11 grams of protein per cup
Cheeses contain about 12 grams of protein per 2 ounces
Cottage cheese, whole
Plain yogurt, whole (*you* sweeten it)
Goat cheese or yogurt (a common fresh goat cheese is called chèvre)
Sheep milk yogurt/cheese
Sheep cheese (Valbreso feta, pecorino Romano)
Raw-milk cheeses (many varieties; several European aged cheeses are raw-milk, such as Gruyère and Asiago)
Kefir or other cultured dairy products

VEGETABLE SOURCES OF PROTEIN:
Beans contain 7 to 15 grams of protein per 3 ounces
Beans are discussed in the carbohydrate chapter (see page 118) because they contain 10 to 20 grams of natural net carbohydrate to acquire the said protein content. The 2:1 ratio of carb to protein makes them a higher protein than grains, but not at all like meats and eggs. For example: 3 ounces of garbanzo beans contain about 8 grams of protein and 20 grams of natural net carbohydrate, whereas an extra large egg has 8 grams of protein and zero carb.

Tofu is a processed, concentrated, soybean product where 80 to 90 percent of the fiber and carbohydrate portion of the bean is removed, while leaving the protein. This is no longer a whole food. As a food is processed and one portion of it is concentrated, there are usually problems. Tofu is likely not nearly as harmful as other ubiquitous processed-food proteins, namely, soy protein isolate. This highly processed soy-derived protein (aka, isolated soy protein) is frequently found in soy milk and protein bars, and as a cheap filler for foods like sliced sandwich meats, some canned tuna, and hot dogs.

SLIGHTLY PROCESSED MEAT/POULTRY:
Slightly processed forms of meat and poultry (e.g., sliced sandwich meats, highly salted meats like ham, and smoked or cured meats like dry sausage should not be used as daily dietary staples, but are useful picnic-style proteins.

NATURAL CURED MEATS:
There are traditional ways to dry and cure meats (including beef jerky). Many butchers offer a traditional biltong-style beef jerky with no preservatives.

SALT-CURED MEATS AND SAUSAGES:
Good-quality ham and traditional salt-cured meats can be found without added preservatives or sugar. Sausages, from turkey, pork, chicken, and lamb, made fresh with simple, non-processed ingredients are available at many full-service butcher shops.

SANDWICH MEATS:
Sandwich meats should be cut right off the roast; the ingredients list should be simple, without cheap added fillers, such as dextrose or soy protein. However, it's important to remember that even the most natural sandwich meats have an unusually high salt content, and should be used in moderation.

The Healthiest Dense Proteins

In my lifelong quest to find the healthiest diet, it is no surprise that I was on the vegetarian train for many years in my twenties. But since my own insulin resistance required that I eat more dense and fatty proteins instead of beans and brown rice, I had to relearn how to purchase and prepare meats. A slow-cooked (braised), bone-in roast is truly the most nutrient-dense form of protein, and now that I have learned how to do it, I find that it's the easiest meal to prepare.

Beef and lamb are the densest of the protein sources. This means that a lot of caloric nutrients are packed into a small space, so you don't need to eat as much to get adequate protein or calories. Chuck roast is about 50 percent fat and 50 percent protein, and 0 percent carbohydrate and fiber; when trimmed, it usually leaves 30 percent fat by weight. Meat portions with 30 percent fat by weight is calorically 50 percent fat. These foods provide sustainable energy, and can be eaten in relatively small volumes to satisfy your nutrient needs

My Take on Vegetarianism

I was a vegetarian in my early twenties. It was early in my career, and at the beginning of my quest for the healthiest diet. The dominant trend seemed valid on the surface, and I relished the I-am-right-about-this attitude. I can now see the incredible holes in the hyped claims of various authorities I read and followed. My clinical vocation is dedicated to helping people find the diet that prevents chronic illness and allows a family to live the longest and healthiest life possible. If I really thought that going vegetarian would help in that direction, I'd be the first to tell you, but the data is just not there. I will not even entertain the thought of veganism, as there is not a single reproducing culture of humans on Earth that is vegan.

There is truth to the studies that found the highest 20 percent of meat eaters in America had more heart disease than the lowest 20 percent, but these studies have been better analyzed, and the processed-meat intake appears to be the kicker. I am obviously no longer vegetarian, and in my experience, people have to eat some animal proteins in order to recover their health and vitality, *especially* those with insulin resistance. Their physical and emotional health improves, and blood tests confirm that their choices are right for them for the long haul.

—Dr. Richard Maurer

While I believe that you should not be in the top 20 percent of people who eat *processed* meat, the demonization of red meat should stop, given the current data. Results from a 2010 study have been consistent with many others that followed: "Consumption of processed meats, but not red meats, is associated with higher incidence of CHD and diabetes mellitus. These results highlight the need for better understanding of potential mechanisms of effects and for particular focus on processed meats for dietary and policy recommendations."[11]

In 2013, researchers studied 450,000 people, and made the following conclusions[12]:

- High consumption of processed meat was related to moderately higher all-cause mortality. Red meat and poultry intake was not associated with mortality.
- Several vegetarian studies did not find increased all-cause mortality among non-vegetarians compared with vegetarians.
- There was consistent association between processed-meat consumption and total mortality, but not between red meat consumption and total mortality.
- There was no statistically significant association of red meat consumption with risk of cancer or cardiovascular mortality.

So what's so bad about *processed* meat? This book is not going to attempt to offer a definitive answer for why processed meat—or any other processed food, for that matter—is harmful to your health. Suffice to say that processing foods with methods that have not been tried or tested over many generations is a risky venture. Traditional cuisine is safer. I don't know the precise variable or set of variables that make processed meat so unhealthy. Is it the preservatives; the excess salt in relation to other mineral nutrients; or the oxidation and degradation of the fats due to excessive handling, transport, and storage times? Is it the packaging materials, or the growing, feeding, or slaughter conditions? Is it the addition of oxidized "pink slime" or other processed food protein to boost the leanness of the final meat product beyond what is normally found on the animal?

Simply stated, I believe that processed food is not healthy, and that includes common sandwich meats and things like "Clucko-Chicken-Bites."

This may sound obvious to many of you, but now conclusive research is on your side.

Healthy Whole Meats

Unprocessed meat includes freshly ground hamburger (not leaner than 85 percent!); whole cuts of meat typically found at a butcher's shop, such as roasts, steaks, lamb cuts, and parts of whole chicken and turkey. The cut should be identifiable as to its source.

How this looks on the table: At a family dining–style restaurant in Tuscany, served up by the acclaimed butcher and chef, Dario Cecchini, I was delighted to see the fatty beef roast sliced thin and immediately set into a lively Italian olive oil bath (a culinary trick to keep the nutritious and flavor-filled juices from escaping the slices of meat). A mouthful of this sublime dish reminded me that a piece of unprocessed beef is not necessarily high protein; most of the calories came from the fats. The spread of fresh vegetables was a tremendous complement, and a little bowl of white beans with olive oil provided a starchy fiber, again with olive oil.

Fish and Shellfish

Fish is a leaner meat, and therefore should be cooked with adequate fats. The fats are less saturated and contain more of the essential EPA ome-ga-3 variety than red meats. Fish is less dense and contains less sinewy fibers; this means that if you have a weaker digestion, you will usually feel better after a fish meal.

Dietary fats with fish: Broil fish with butter or olive oil. Serve the fish with a lemon and crème fraîche dip. The addition of fats to the meal will allow fish to become a sustainable protein. Oily fish such as eel and small fish such as anchovies, sardines, and mackerel all provide a tremendous supply of the healthy essential fats. Easy and convenient canned fish, such as bone-in sardines, offer a tremendous source of mineral nutrition, with a calcium supply equivalent to a glass of milk (but unlike milk, contain no simple carbohydrate).

Chicken and Other Poultry

Chicken, turkey, and duck, unlike red meats, have a distinct separation of fats and protein. The white meat tends to be low in fat, and therefore low in essential fats and fat-soluble vitamins. The skin holds the fatty nutrients. The vast majority of the vitamin and mineral content of chicken, like other meats and fish, is tied up in the bones and connective tissue. Broth and gravy made out of the juices that come from cooking the whole bird are where the real powerhouse of nutrition comes from.

Blood Code Favorite: Whole Roast Chicken

Purchase a whole chicken. Rub with olive oil, salt, pepper, and any herbs you like, fresh or dry. Place in a roasting pan with a cover; a clay pot is remarkably good for this, but foil works too. Roast for four hours at 275 degrees F., or closer to two hours at 375 degrees. In the last hour, throw whatever root veggies you like around the roast to cook and absorb the juices (carrots, onions, turnips, potatoes).

Any leftover meat will be tomorrow's chicken salad, or meat for a soup.

Broth: After everyone eats the meal, leftover skin, meat scraps, and bones can be scraped into a pot of water; boil for a few hours, adding vegetable scraps, too. A pressure cooker shortens the cooking time needed to get the nutrients out of the bones and veggies. No need to worry about "germs," as the long boiling sterilizes the broth.

In France, rotisserie chicken is quite popular, but unlike the American version I see in supermarkets, the French have potatoes in a tray underneath the chickens, catching the nutrient-rich drippings. The potato is now a vehicle to get those nutrients back into your diet.

Nutrients are "hidden" in the bones and organs: People in most cultures around the world eat organ meats, including liver, bone marrow, heart, kidney, and tripe. Yet most "Westernized" people reflexively exclaim "Gross!" at the mere thought of it. Broth is a tremendous way to extract nutrients from bones, organs, and cartilage, with very little culinary objection. The broth can then be used as the liquid to cook rice, or to make a soup or stew.

Protein and Reduced Food Cravings

Something to consider when you are hankering for something to eat: Is it hunger, or a craving? If it is a craving, lack of adequate protein in the prior day or days may be the trigger. You can bet the $60 billion weight-loss market has funded some studies into food cravings, and one of the few proven dietary additions is protein. Protein does trigger satiety, a condition that helps you feel satisfied and eat less in subsequent meals on that day. This effect is remarkably significant when researchers compare food cravings in people that eat a protein-rich breakfast versus a carbohydrate breakfast.[13]

An exhaustive review of high-protein diets was published in 2004, and subsequent studies confirm the results. High protein in these diets varies widely, from 100 grams per day to 300 grams per day. Three hundred grams of protein did not garner more impressive results than 150 grams. Your Blood Code Diet requires 0.5 to 1 gram of protein per pound of lean body mass; the upper half of your target range is adequate to gain the weight management, mood, and satiety benefits of a high-protein diet.[14]

Dietary protein in my diet . . .

I roast a whole chicken once a week, which typically provides us with two nights' worth of meals. On the other nights we have lamb, slow-cooked pork or beef roast, freshly ground hamburger, and fish/shellfish. My one to two eggs, 350 mornings per year, provide 7 to 14 grams of protein to start my day. Lunch is leftovers, which puts the pressure on getting the dinner protein right. In a pinch, about weekly, I can rely on the canned salmon and sardines that are in the cabinet.

Four Dietary Principles

I can see the 1930s *Little Rascals* episode now. A child goes to grab something to eat from the kitchen, and the message is clear: "Not now; you'll spoil your dinner." At a young age, kids were taught not to eat between meals.

Where do you get your guidelines now? Where is the beacon of how to eat if not shining clearly through afternoon television? Well, here you go.

Principle #1: Don't overfill your plate or overstock your kitchen.

In his 2006 book *Mindless Eating*, Brian Wansink performs various experiments to show that we humans actually have a pathetic capacity to self-regulate. The size of the portion we see on our plate strongly influences the quantity we eat. Simply put, if you put less on the plate, or in the serving bowl, less will be consumed. He went one better in his experiments and invited people to cook dinner themselves. One group had access to big bottles of sauce and pasta, and the other, more reasonably sized packages of ingredients. You guessed it: The group with the larger packages of ingredients made 23 percent more food and ate it all, just the same.

Americans have the biggest refrigerators in the world. I suggest that if someone did a study, there would be a direct correlation between food storage capacity and food intake.

Principle #2: Avoid processed foods, including artificial and natural flavors, artificial sweeteners, and the like.

Sorry to say it again, but processed foods are problematic to your health. Dr. David Kessler, a man with a remarkable résumé, wrote a book called *The End of Overeating*. The title implies that the solution to overeating is found in his book, but it primarily provides another answer to the important "Why are you overweight?" question. He presents the tension between the food manufacturing industry, which works hard to "unlock the code of crave-ability," and your health, which requires you to exercise temperance. You need to know and practice the adage "Enough is enough," which is made more difficult by the prevalence of food chemicals that try to push you to eat more and more. Overeating is, in part, a conditioned response to food stimulus in the mouth. The food industry has no shortage of chemicals that stimulate all sorts of alluring experiences in your mind and body. Study after study have shown that processed food compromises your health. Dr. Kessler's work is yet another pin in the balloon of food additives and processed foods.

Principle #3: Rituals are okay; more variety is not necessarily better.

There was a study in England in the 1990s that discovered people who ate less variety at breakfast ate fewer calories and reported more satiety. The fewer ingredients in a meal, and the more your body senses familiar flavors and textures, the better you can self-regulate how much to eat.

Another study did the same thing with alcohol. For years, people blamed their hangover on the fact that they mixed different alcohols in a night. It turned out, when studied under controlled circumstances, that people who stayed with one kind of drink got no more intoxicated than people who mixed drinks, *but,* people who mixed different kinds of drinks drank more than they reported. When your mouth and body experience something new, there is a subconscious response in your brain that says, "Ooh, I want more of *that.*"

Again, the simplicity of the Mediterranean diet seems apt. Although less familiar to me, I am sure the same would be true for those accustomed to the diets of Thailand or Japan. The quality of fresh ingredients is kept simple in both recipe and preparation. The local food and slow food movements present great opportunities for Americans to rediscover their roots and take their diets back to simple, more local ingredients. The now-famous chef Alice Waters, in her California bioregional restaurant, Chez Panisse, has rightfully been acknowledged for her mastery of simple preparation of fresh, local ingredients. Less may be more in this case.

Principle #4: Eat no more than three times per day.

In surveys around the globe, people in every other country eat less frequently than in America. It's commonplace for these people to eat just two and a half meals per day. A study done in Greece in 2007 showed that postmenopausal women who ate more frequently had more body fat. The researchers not so succinctly summarized: "Frequent eating predisposes women after menopause to a higher energy intake by increasing food stimuli and rendering it more difficult for them to control energy balance."[15] Allow me to offer my take: If you eat too often, you will eat too much.

The American recommendation to eat more frequent meals has only been post-1970, when low-fat foods mistakenly became the federal recommendation, thus making it more difficult to make it four to six hours without eating. The American theory of eating more-frequent low-fat meals has helped to create the overweight, over-diabetic culture that you see today.

When should you eat your biggest meal? In short, it doesn't matter. It is clear that those who eat breakfast are more likely to perform better on tests, have more stable moods, and have fewer "bad" habits, such as smoking. So skipping breakfast is risky. Most places in the world have a smaller morning meal. Weight management does not differ whether the midday or evening meal is larger.

If you can't make it between meals without snacking, or you're dissatisfied, add more fats to the prior meal and ensure that you had ample soluble fiber from the "Staple Carbohydrates" (see page 114—118).

As with any rule, it can be broken. Some athletes will require 3,000 to 5,000 calories per day during peak training. This requires a fourth meal to sustain the demanding caloric load.

Dietary Myths Removed

It ain't what you don't know that gets you into trouble. It's what you know for sure that just ain't so.
—Mark Twain

Every day, in my practice, I hear misplaced confidence from patients when they claim, "I don't ever have salt," or "I reduced my carbs by switching to whole grains." I could probably fill a book with dietary myths and the truths behind them, but here are five that I think are worth mentioning:

Five Dietary Myths:

1) Whole grains are healthier than refined grains.
2) Dietary saturated fats are harmful.
3) Raw food is healthier than cooked food.
4) It is better to eat smaller meals, and more frequently.
5) Salt intake is bad for you.

Revealing the Truth:

#1—Whole grains are high-carb foods that contain virtually the same carb content as the more-refined version of the same grain.

People with insulin resistance are wrongly advised to switch to whole grains; the difference in carb content is negligible—41 versus 44 grams of carb in 1 cup of brown versus white rice. The nutrient content difference is negligible, too. There is a little extra insoluble fiber content in whole grains, but that doesn't matter much, as soluble fiber is the kind that offers the most health benefits.

The "whole grain is healthy" myth exists, I believe, because of two other problems. Processed foods with refined white flour usually contain added refined sugar. The sugars are more responsible for health problems than the white flour. The second problem? Refined-flour products can be eaten faster, meaning, more is consumed; overeating is therefore the problem, not the flour color.

Whole grains have the same amount of soluble fiber as more-refined grains. Whole-wheat flour and brown rice have the same soluble fiber content as white flour and white rice, respectively. There are a couple extra grams of insoluble fiber per cup in the whole version, and minimal nutrient differences. The process of removing the indigestible husk from the grain is thousands of years old, and, as you can imagine, helps the food starch become more digestible and less irritating. The healthiest and best-tolerated fiber ratio is about 1:1, soluble to insoluble, which is what's found in most vegetables, fruits, and legumes.

The processed-food industry jumped on this myth and loaded extra insoluble fiber from "whole grains" into boxed cereal and cereal bars. If you ate a half-ounce of sand, that would equal 16 grams of insoluble fiber. Eating sand for fiber sounds absurd, but it's not unlike the 15 grams of insoluble fiber added to a processed breakfast cereal. Additional insoluble fiber is used in foods to inflate the health claims, not to improve your nutrition.[16] Sugar-laden, "whole-grain" boxed cereal is unhealthy, regardless of what the label states.

Foods with natural soluble fiber provide a decreased breast cancer risk, not insoluble fiber. In a remarkably large study through the US National Institutes of Health, soluble fiber was shown to be more effective in controlling blood glucose, insulin, and insulin-like growth factors, thereby lowering the risk of breast cancer. The researchers went further to state that total fat intake was not a risk factor for cancer.[17] Vegetables added to a diet of white rice is better than a switch to brown rice, with more soluble fiber and less irritating to digestion. Just count the carb content of the grain, regardless of its color.

#2—Saturated fats are not the problem.

The vilification of saturated fat is unsustainable. Period. To have passed this moral judgment upon a food is a shame of science. Saturated fats from traditional sources are an essential part of your Blood Code Diet. A diet that is lower in carbs and higher in fats allows your body to burn fats for energy more effectively.

Different food sources of saturated fats offer unique cooking and nutritional benefits, including butter; cultured cream; coconut oil; chicken, duck, or goose fat; and pork fat (lard).

Historically and appropriately, dietary fats are revered. In Jewish tradition, rendered chicken or goose fat is called *schmaltz*. According to an old saying, if a baby was born to a very fortunate and well-off family, that child "was born into the schmaltz pot." The French have another saying that displays how quality dietary fats are to be regarded: "crème de la crème." The higher-fat cream that comes to the top of raw cream as it cultures is truly the "best of the best."

Saturated fats have been vindicated. Modern comprehensive analysis of the Framingham Study data—the very data that caused the false blame to be laid on dietary saturated fat, thirty years ago—has revealed that no such blame was scientifically warranted.

The lead investigator from the Harvard team, Dr. Dariush Mozaffarian, summarized the importance of this meta-analysis study: "This is pretty important on a policy level. It's naturally assumed that lowering saturated fat is good for the heart, but that's not what the evidence shows." Furthermore, based upon the meta-analysis, he concludes, "There was no significant evidence that dietary saturated fat is associated with an increased risk of coronary heart disease or cardiovascular disease."[18]

Further studies, again by the same noted researcher, have pointed the finger of cardiovascular disease risk toward processed foods and the high-carb intake that typically replaces reduced fat intake.[19][20]

Of course, when people reduce saturated fats, they will replace the calories with something like carbs. Unsaturated fats come with unique cancer and heart disease risks when eaten in place of saturated fats. A very recent study found that in men who had already had a heart attack, substituting dietary linoleic acid, such as from sunflower, safflower, or corn oil, in place of saturated fats increased the rates of death from all causes, including both coronary heart disease and cardiovascular disease.[21]

#3—Traditional food preparation, including cooking, is necessary for human digestion; raw food is not healthier.

Vegetables are great sources of minerals, but these nutrients are better absorbed when the food source is cooked. A serving of broccoli or dark leafy greens has a glass of milk's worth of calcium, but the calcium and nutrient minerals are part of the structural integrity of the vegetable, and are trapped inside the stiff fibers. When cooked, the fibers release the nutrients for your digestion. Heat does not degrade minerals, and some vitamins gain potency when the food is cooked.[22]

"Enzymes" are traditionally found in fermented foods, such as kimchi, sauerkraut, or other fermented vegetables. Many foods historically were "cooked" by soaking them in vinegar or acids, such as pickled vegetables, coleslaw, or cured meats. When the acidic vinegar or lemon juice is added to a food, it breaks down the cell walls, allowing your body to digest the available nutrients. So fermenting and culturing is really a kind of "cooking."

True, if you chew well, and have a strong acidic stomach to digest and break down the food, your body will "cook" the vegetable for you in your 100-degree acidic stomach. But with small teeth and a bacteria-less stomach, humans require some preparation to release the nutrients that are trapped in the fibrous parts of the plant or animal.[23]

#4—There is no traditional culture on Earth that eats more than three times per day.

Once saturated fat was wrongly demonized in the 1970s and 1980s, people who adopted the low-fat diet found themselves hungry every three hours.

Physiologically, your digestive tract requires about four to six hours or longer to move one meal from the stomach to the end of the absorptive small intestine. It is best to add food to the stomach only after the prior meal has completed the absorptive process. This allows adequate time for digestion and absorption of nutrients.

What about smaller meals? Smaller *volume*, yes. Higher-fat meals give you more nutrition in a smaller volume. Your stomach will stretch less, and less insulin will be released. Your Blood Code Diet should include high-fat meals that allow you to "make it" between meals without the need to snack.

#5—Real salt is not the culprit; processed food, once again, is the culprit.

Salt is essential for every function in your body. Dietary recommendations for salt intake fixate on avoidance, not on how much you *should* have. Your daily intake should be about 2,400 mg—approximately 1 teaspoon of fine- to medium-grain salt. If you begin your diet with whole, unprocessed foods, you will need to add and ensure adequate salt intake. No study has ever found the high blood pressure / salt connection from the use of salt in the home kitchen or at the table.

So why has *everyone* been told to reduce their salt intake? Institutions carelessly treat us all as though we, as individuals, are the statistical average. Let me explain. If you include people who eat highly processed foods: One slice of processed luncheon meat has 500 to 600 mg salt in one slice, so, without including the bag of chips, a loaded Italian sandwich with eight slices of processed meat contains over 4,000 mg of salt. This group will thus consume more than 6,000 mg of salt per day. There are other people who do *not* consume processed sandwich meats on a daily basis, and they are ingesting less than 2,000 mg of salt per day.

Statistics show that Americans take in an average of about 4,000 mg of salt per day. Researchers surmise that if this average was lowered by 1,500 mg, there would be less high blood pressure. So authorities told everyone to reduce their salt intake by 1,500 mg per day. This turns out to be inadequate for those people who consume 6,000 mg per day, and too much of a salt restriction for people who consume 2,000 mg per day. The people on either end of the bell curve will be worse off if they follow these salt-reduction recommendations.

The Blood Code is about helping *you* address your unique dietary and nutritional needs in a way that is likely to improve your own life and health. Most of us are not well served by following a list of dietary guidelines that are designed to treat a mathematical average.

If you start with whole, unprocessed meats, vegetables, starches, and fats, you will need to add the 2,400 mg of salt yourself. Lay out a teaspoon of salt and make sure it is gone by the end of the day. Research has also shown that as people exercise more, the connection between high blood pressure and salt intake evaporates. If you have hypertension, by all means, avoid processed foods, but do not "over-restrict" salt at home; it is a necessary mineral/electrolyte nutrient.

Step Five: Add The Blood Code Fitness Principles

Exercise should be regarded as tribute to the heart.
—Gene Tunney, heavyweight boxing legend

At this point, you have gained some valuable insight about yourself through Steps One to Three. The dietary habits discussed in Step Four start the ball rolling toward your rightful and healthy metabolism. Your fitness lifestyle is the other side of the action-coin. You might fully recover your insulin resistance with dietary changes alone, but over time—many years, perhaps— you will ultimately need to self-prescribe some essential fitness habits.

Over the past twenty years, scientific literature has been loaded with useful and practical information about the effects of different types of exercise. There has also been a glut of technologies that take you away from a physically active lifestyle. There is a bright side to this confluence: Studies have shown that exercise does not need to take a long time. You can practice long runs, and that may help you to become a better long-distance runner; however, it won't make you more insulin-sensitive. Your metabolism benefits from bursts of a different kind of exercise. Headlines have once again dumbed down the message, and claims of "3-minute abs" and a "5-minute workout" are misleading. The Blood Code Fitness Principles are designed to get your metabolism moving in the right direction for the rest of your life.

What have you learned about yourself?

If You're Insulin-Resistant

Men and women with type 2 diabetes or prediabetes are usually told to exercise because it will help to control their blood sugar. The word *help* is pretty weak—as though exercise is something that can be done on the side to help you feel a little better. Research has shown that exercise is more than your backup plan; it should be front and center in your daily life. Effective fitness habits play a primary and foundational role in your healthy metabolism and disease prevention.

If you have any of level of insulin resistance, your body has proven its efficiency at storing and leaving behind extra fats and sugars. Therefore, you need to exercise in a way that trains your body to burn and utilize the stored fats, glucose, and glycogen on a daily (and hourly) basis. The Fitness Principles that follow will condition and train your body to use what it has stored; the result will be a remarkable improvement in your energy and metabolism.

If You Need to Lower Insulin

Not all types of exercise can transform you from disease-prone insulin resistance to healthier insulin sensitivity. Your muscles take up the bulk of the glucose in your body. Basic aerobic exercise, like a jog or a walk that lasts at least 30 minutes, does result in benefits: Blood sugars will get utilized, and will therefore be lowered; your HDL will increase, and your blood pressure decrease. So it's clearly better than nothing.

But if you have insulin resistance, *you will not turn your metabolism around with mere aerobic exercise.* You will not reverse the insulin-resistant trend that is sending you toward weight gain, lipid problems, and countless disease risks. Furthermore, if aerobic exercise is extended for long periods of time, regular bouts of greater than one hour at a time, your muscle mass will tend to decrease, leaving you more sluggish metabolically and more insulin-resistant.

This needs to be said again: An hour on the treadmill will burn calories, sure, but it can actually *lower* your muscle mass and make you even *more* insulin-resistant over time. Your goal is to maintain or gain your muscle mass as compared to your body fat. This is why skin-fold calipers are superior to a scale. If you lose fat while exercising regularly, your body will likely build a more metabolically active muscle. The scale won't show weight loss, but the calipers and your clothes will show fat loss. Your Blood Code fitness habits should support and move you toward a metabolically active body. Your Blood Code Progress Panel will clearly and objectively mark your fitness success by showing a lower TG:HDL ratio and a lower HOMA-IR—the closer to 1, the better. With regular, appropriate exercise in your life, you should have a HOMA-IR of 1 or less.

To Initiate Exercise While on Prescription Metformin

Exercise works better than metformin to control blood sugars,[1] yet metformin can interfere with exercise performance. Metformin is a drug that prevents the release of sugar that is stored in your muscles and liver. Does metformin lower your blood sugar if it is high? Yes. However, it accomplishes this not by getting rid of the excessive sugar in your body tissues, but by locking the door so the glucose is also prevented from being released.

In one study, the drug metformin was linked to higher heart rates and more subjective fatigue under exercise conditions. Researchers absurdly cited this as a reason people on metformin might need to work out less strenuously.[2] Free fatty acids, a fuel source that funds most activities in your body, are 10 to 20 percent lower in those who are taking metformin.

But since regular strenuous exercise can improve insulin resistance better than metformin,[3] it is preferable to adjust the latter. I hate to say it, but your doctor will be reluctant to reduce your metformin because he/she assumes that you are more likely to stick with popping a pill than complying with a regular exercise routine. So even though exercise is a superior therapy, the medical advice you receive could be based upon your presumed failure. I know that you are not the statistical average; you are a motivated individual who has taken a few big steps to reach this far into this book. Your success is up to you, and I'll try to guide you along as you include more exercise into each day of your week. Discuss your metformin dosage and any possible dosage adjustments with your doctor, and check your results with the contents of the Progress Panel within three to four months.

The Hypothyroid Trait

If, through Step One (Thyroid), you discovered that you have a hypothyroid trait, this means that your body is a slow burner at rest. Did you hear that? *At rest.* Exercise, done in a way that is described here in Step Five, partially replaces and trumps the metabolism that thyroid hormones provide. In fact, studies have clearly shown that non-hypothyroid individuals have substantially lower thyroid hormones after vigorous exercise, especially if that exercise is done in a warm environment. This makes perfect sense for self-preservation. Thyroid activity is not required to generate your baseline metabolism if your vigorous exercise has generated heat in your cells.[4]

If you express a hypothyroid trait, your metabolism is slow on the days off. You will need to practice The Blood Code Fitness Principles *daily* in order to keep that active metabolism and the energy you want, and deserve. Again, remember the good news: It doesn't need to be a long time; 20 minutes is plenty if your activity is vigorous enough.

The Four Fitness Principles

The Blood Code Fitness Principles

1) Exercise on an empty stomach.
2) Exercise strenuously and vigorously.
3) Engage many muscle groups whenever possible.
4) Vary your heart rate throughout.

Principle #1: Do not eat before exercise.

In the Step Four chapter, "Adjust Your Blood Code Diet," you learned that your body prefers to use the calories that it's already wearing—your stored fats and sugars. For the subsequent hours, your body works to replenish what has been broken down. For lean athletes, it will be important to feed your body a protein-rich meal after a vigorous workout, to help repair and replace the necessary muscle and supportive structures of your body. But most people are not functioning at their lowest tolerable body fat percentage (near "Too Low" on the Step Two charts; see page 70). If you have not recently eaten prior to exercising, your insulin will be lower; and if your insulin is kept low during your workouts, you will effectively burn fats more readily. As you move toward a lower insulin level throughout the day, your body fat and circulating triglycerides will more readily be utilized to provide sustained energy both at exercise and at rest.

Is this like fasting? Maybe, a little. In the 1990s, researchers reported that calorically deprived mice lived longer than their better-fed kin. This headline led to a plethora of speculation and personal trials, as people in their later years began eating "like birds" in hopes that they might live like old mice. Intermittent fasting was all the rage. Research now clarifies that the reduction in your circulating insulin level is likely a key mechanism toward an extended life span. Low insulin levels have been associated with people who live for more than ninety years. Your net insulin sensitivity is an important marker in your Blood Code success toward longevity. As you begin to practice the Fitness Principles on a regular basis, your Blood Code Panels should reflect an improvement in your insulin sensitivity. Your HOMA-IR should be as close to 1 as possible, and if it's lower than 1, that's good news for now and a *long* time to come![5678]

Principle #2: Your exercise routine needs to be vigorous; not longer, just more strenuous.

A landmark study back in 2008 by a Norwegian team of researchers opened with the sentence, "Individuals with the metabolic syndrome are three times more likely to die from heart disease than healthy counterparts." Okay, did you hear that? If you are one of the 40 to 50 percent that express some insulin resistance, you should be listening. The researchers conclude, "The current study suggests that exercise in general, and AIT [Aerobic Interval Training] in particular, is partly or fully able to reverse metabolic syndrome . . . Guidelines calling for 30 minutes of exercise of moderate intensity may be too general for this population."[9]

Vigorous physical activity improves insulin sensitivity. I'm saying this again because it is important.

In another study that specifically looked at insulin sensitivity, people with elevated fasting blood sugars were given mild, moderate, and intense weight routines. Blood glucose improved in all groups, although those who did the most intense exercise earned the greatest insulin sensitivity, and the benefit was seen more than twenty-four hours after the workout. Insulin sensitivity means there is a reduction in blood sugar along with a reduction in overall insulin. Vigorous exercise, in this particular study, was reached by performing four sets of eight upper and lower body-strength exercises at high intensity (85 percent of one-repetition maximum, for those who like to know the details). The participants did less than ten repetitions of each exercise back-to-back, with little rest in between. The workout lasted about 20 minutes.[10]

More-recent studies continue to show the benefits of weight and strength training, and this knowledge is eroding the faith we used to have in the benefits of long, sustained aerobic exercise. But of course, aerobic versus non-aerobic exercise is not an either-or. Maintaining a well-conditioned heart through aerobic exercise is exceptionally healthful, but benefits fall short if that aerobic exercise does not vary in intensity and does not push the muscles to "full contraction," like strength training does.

Even big, clumsy, authoritative organizations have responded to the convincing evidence about exercise intensity. The American Heart Association now states that "Short bursts of high-intensity exercise, rather than longer spells of moderate-intensity exercise, may improve the health of people with metabolic syndrome [insulin resistance]."

The research that shows the most successful metabolic outcomes indicates that supervision by a trained individual is key. A book is terribly limited in its ability to teach fitness, a mere description of exercises would be unhelpful. I encourage you to personally see a qualified trainer who is familiar with the Fitness Principles that follow. Visit TheBloodCode.com to find the current resources that are being developed for you to get the most efficient and effective metabolic recovery instruction possible.

Principle #3: Engage many muscle groups during exercise.

Virtually all sit-down exercise equipment forces you to use only one muscle group in a linear motion without engaging the core muscles of balance. This will not work for you. Those of you who have some insulin resistance or slower thyroid need to create a fitness practice that is as metabolically active as possible. Insulin resistance, remember, is not some diseased state; it is a state of remarkable efficiency. Your efficient metabolism has evolved in an environment full of "inefficient" activities.

My ancestors did not get water by turning a faucet; they needed to haul water (eight pounds per gallon) by hand from a central well, perhaps a couple of miles away. The efficiency in my current life is staggering. I can get my mail with the click of a keyboard, and deliver water with the turn of a faucet to ten different places around my house. I am peripheral insulin-resistant, which means my metabolism is hyperefficient. I need to exercise in a way that is actually more *in*efficient; that is, I have to strenuously engage many different muscle groups in every type of exercise.

So forget the old exercise goal of "isolating a muscle group"; in contrast, you are to engage an extra muscle group. Trainers encourage people in this direction for other reasons. If you have exercised and toned the surrounding muscles of support and your core muscles of stability, you are less prone to injury, your balance is better, and you get a more-complete workout in a shorter time period.

Principle #4: Vary your heart rate throughout your exercise routine.

I grew up in a marathon-running family in the 1970s and early '80s. Marathons are the archetypal aerobic activity: The runner tries to control his or her target heart rate, keeping it low and steady throughout the run. Those who can keep their heart rate lower have a competitive advantage. Over time, long-distance runners develop a slow resting heart rate, to compensate for the long-sustained increased heart rate from hours of continuous running.

A slow resting heart rate used to be the mark of heart health, but newer and better research offers a different story. Even back in the 1930s there were signs that "good conditioning" was not about slowing the heart down. During this decade, the Swedish cross-country running team famously improved their performance through an interval training program called *fartlek*—"speed play" in Swedish. I don't think a fitness program would succeed today with a name like *fartlek;* therefore, terms like *interval training, cross training, circuit training,* and *high-intensity training* are used to describe the similar practice of "short bursts of more intense activity with interspersed periods of active recovery."

Convincing research now shows that "heart rate recovery," a measure of how quickly and how much your heartbeat (pulse) slows back down from a prior effort, is the best mark of your cardiometabolic health.[11][12]

You were born with a healthy heart rate recovery, but, like many things, if you don't use it, you'll lose it. Watch kids free-play in the outdoors, and you'll notice that they exhibit a "go until you can't, rest until you can" pattern—a very natural and innate exercise style. Fortunately, it's never too late to relearn!

An impressive it's-not-too-late study was done on older people who already had a condition of severe heart disease, and they displayed substantial improvement with their heart rate recovery when they participated in a circuit-type exercise program for at least one hour, three days per week (with supervision), over a twelve-week period. One of the researchers, Leslie Cho, MD, commented on the results of the study, and I couldn't say it any better myself: "There's no medicine that can do that, especially in terms of mortality. . . . If we had a medicine that could make this dramatic an impact, it would be the blockbuster drug of the century."[13]

Your Blood Code Fitness Principles in Action

There is more than one way to exercise for insulin sensitivity; as long as your exercise follows the Blood Code Fitness Principles, you will get there. You need to know what will keep you motivated, because this is not about what you're going to do for the next couple of months—it's about the rest of your life.

If you already have a regular exercise routine: You might already have a walking group, or regularly bike to work. While this activity is a step in the right direction, it does not correct your excessive metabolic efficiency. While it is easy to apply Principle #2, the others require a little creativity. Janet did a great job of adding two of the Fitness Principles to her regular walk, effectively correcting her insulin resistance (see her case study below).

Success from Small Changes in Exercise
Janet L., sixty-three years old

Janet had mild insulin resistance that she was able to correct with pretty minor changes to her exercise. She had been on the Blood Code Diet for two years, yet her sugars remained slightly elevated.

Janet had a walking routine with friends six days per week, three miles per walk. Habit and social support are critical, so instead of changing her routine, she used 3-pound dumbbells in her hands. At intervals throughout the walk, she did a few sets of overhead presses, curls, and side lifts with the dumbbell weight. At the end of the walk, she did 5 minutes of moderately strenuous core exercises.

Principle #2: She engaged muscles that used to be "asleep at the wheel" during her walk.
Principle #3: Walking is not strenuous; she added that element with weights.

"I can't believe that is all I needed to do. It doesn't take any more time, and I can feel that I've gotten stronger." And the numbers show it too. *

Panel Test Date	4/11/10	5/5/12	8/10/12*
Cholesterol, mg/dL	204	199	190
Triglyceride, mg/dL	90	98	64
HDL, mg/dL	48	48	59
TG:HDL ratio	1.9	2.0	1.1
HgbA1C %	6.2	6.0	5.5
Fasting glucose, mg/dL	108	102	89
Fasting insulin, uIU/mL	10	10	7
HOMA−IR	2.7	2.5	1.5

Now, I could rain on Janet's parade and explain that she might need to make more exercise effort in ten years, but for now, her efforts are working well. As you age, you have to expend *more* effort to maintain the same muscle mass you had when you were younger.

Tips for Fitness Success

By my mid-forties, I had a list of excuses at the ready when it came to exercise: a torn cartilage in my knee, scoliosis, an extra lumbar vertebrae, and a past broken tailbone. A well-motivated older patient of mine aptly said to me that while these may be reasons, there are no excuses. What it took was a couple of visits to an athletically attuned physical therapist and some personalized instruction from a qualified trainer to provide me with the skills I needed to work out smarter. I don't need any of the excuses anymore, and have since effectively reduced my insulin resistance by following my own prescribed fitness guidelines.

Here are some other tips that patients have found useful over the years.

- Find a buddy.
- Prevent excuses.
- Do what you can.
- Appreciate and build on measurable success.

If you do better with a group, find one: Fitness condition and obesity are contagious. If you have a buddy with a positive attitude and fitness lifestyle, you're in good company. When you exercise with others, you're more likely to succeed, both long- and short-term. Some people do fine with solo exercise habits; others need the extra motivation. Know yourself, and find the setting that works best to regularly apply the four Fitness Principles into your life.

If you have an injury or condition that requires special consideration: A qualified physical therapist can provide treatment of a condition to get you "back into the game," but from there, you'll need to take it a step further. You need to move from the passive treatments that have you lying on a table to the active exercises that are usually the domain of a sports trainer with a strong understanding of fitness rehab. After an injury or undergoing pain of any kind, it is all too easy to make the excuse that you can't do something. Get some activities going so you can regularly practice the Blood Code Fitness Principles. If you feel stuck, you may need a more-creative definition of exercise. A proper trainer or physical or occupational therapist will help you to avoid excuses.

Do what you can, when you can. Daily! "Not having time" is a cop-out. Prior to 2000, most research condoned the common practice of 30 minutes of continuous exercise. But evidence is mounting that you can change your metabolism in just 10 minutes, done two or three times per day. One study applied moderately intense aerobic exercise on three occasions lasting only 10 minutes each, spread throughout the day. It worked better than 30 minutes of sustained activity. You will have lower blood pressure and be healthier doing this type of workout, even though you may not be an athlete.[14] On days that you "don't have time" for one of your 20- to 30-minute routines, do something . . . anything. If you have the overly efficient metabolism in your Blood Code, your activity must become a daily life habit.

Build on your success. Metabolic fitness is not some location or thing you attain. It is an experience that is only in context with your current diet, lifestyle, and habits. Build a lifestyle of exercise not because you will *get* something out of it, but because of who you will *become*.

Assess the Success of Your Blood Code Fitness Habits

If your Blood Code Progress Panel continues to show insulin resistance, you will, of course, need to reevaluate your dietary guidelines and address your appropriate carbohydrate range. You will also need to be smarter when you "Exercise the Principles." A 30-minute circuit is one of the most proven ways to lower insulin resistance, but this kind of exercise is, by nature, strenuous.

It is probably true that everyone benefits from interval-type exercise, but insulin-resistant people are guaranteed to get the most out of it. Many exercise studies have implemented different exercise strategies for people with insulin resistance, type 2 diabetes, weight problems, and high blood pressure. The most successful of them all use a similar type of fitness routine: a circuit of six to eight resistance exercises that are repeated up to four times over a 30-minute period. Simple, right?

As exercise becomes more strenuous, *how* you do it is as important as *what* you do—especially as you engage more muscle groups. Proper instruction is paramount, so find a qualified trainer. Many trainers and personal fitness studios can help you to develop a program that works for you to practice the Fitness Principles outlined here. Your trainer should be familiar with the principles; there are resources available for both you and your health-care professionals at TheBloodCode.com.

Measure your progress; it's not about your weight: Resistance will make you stronger, less prone to injury, and more metabolically active. The improvement and maintenance of your muscle mass is probably more important now than it was when you were weaker and scrawnier in your youth. Once again, this brings me to the conversation of weight as a poor metric for success. To measure your success, weight is not an adequate marker.

I can't believe that I'm saying you shouldn't exercise for weight loss. The weight-loss product and services industry in America is worth $60 billion. Why wouldn't I want to be a part of that?

Because it's not about me.

It's about you, and what really works. When it comes to your health and longevity, your intention is as important as what you do. Studies repeatedly show that if weight loss is your primary motive, you are the most likely to fail over time. So why, then, is weight loss the primary motivational goal for so many? Because of ever-present myths about what fitness does for you.

Let's crack four of the most tenacious of exercise myths.

Fitness and exercise in my own life . . .

People sometimes say, "You're so lucky that you enjoy exercise." They don't get it. I enjoy how I feel after I exercise; I enjoy living with a body that is as physically adept as possible. But when I wake up and face the daily two-mile run, I don't say, "Oh goody, I get to go run now." I just do it—and the "goody" comes later.

In my early forties, even as a runner, I was expressing insulin resistance, due in part to my low muscle mass and my toast and fruit for breakfast. I don't just run long-distance anymore; five days a week I go about one to two miles, with intervals of all-out sprints. I am done running within 15 to 20 minutes, and then I mix in another 5 to 20 minutes (I fit in what I can, but I always do *something*) of more strenuous exercises I have been taught with bands, balls, a dumbbell, and my body weight. I also use the old-fashioned pull-up bar. Exercising effectively resolves my stress and anxiousness, so I feel better when I've been active.

Since I started doing less running and more strenuous exercise in my 30-minute time frame, I am stronger and less insulin-resistant in my late forties—a good way to enter the second half of my life.

—Dr. Richard Maurer

Fitness Myths Removed

Like your diet, everyone has an opinion about fitness. Recent research has done a fine job of poking holes into many of the preconceived beliefs about exercise. Let's debunk four of the most ubiquitous of these fitness myths:

Four Fitness Myths:

1) Your weight should reduce as your fitness improves.
2) Exercise machines and activity graphs measure calories burned.
3) If you work out your abs, you will reduce belly fat.
4) Stretching prevents injuries.

Revealing the Truth:

Myth #1: In my practice I have seen many people who stopped an exercise program because it "didn't work" in terms of losing weight. An effective fitness habit will help you to build a leaner and more muscular body, and studies continue to confirm that if you maintain regular fitness activity, you will have less heart disease, dementia[15], and chronic disease. With renewed health and strength from a good fitness habit, you will have better blood sugar, less stroke risk, better energy, and clearer thinking. You'll also live longer and be less prone to injury, and be able to fit into a smaller size and have less body fat. But alas, you may not weigh less on a scale.

As you live within your Blood Code, weight loss *will* occur if it's appropriate for you, but weight is not the true barometer of your health and longevity; your Blood Code Panel results and skin-fold caliper measurements will better mark that path.

J. Eric Oliver's 2005 book, *Fat Politics: The Real Story Behind America's Obesity Epidemic,* highlights in convincing detail how the pursuit of weight loss is not only a lost effort institutionally, but probably harmful to your health. If your weight is to improve, it should be through fat loss and health gain. Your fitness goal is to become more insulin-sensitive and burn more fats as energy. You can retest your Blood Code Panel to ensure that you are on the road toward a healthier and happier future.[16]

Myth #2: You can't accurately predict the number of carbs burned while doing a certain activity. A cardio machine spits out a number related to the energy that *it* is experiencing, not you. There are many variables to how much energy *you* expend doing the activity. One of the most prominent is the amount of lean body muscle fibers involved in the activity. Remember to practice Fitness Principle #3—to engage as many muscle groups as possible. This leads to a cruel truth about your physical condition and energy burned: Despite the higher weight of obesity, a leaner person with less body fat actually burns more energy doing the same activity.

It's not all disheartening, although I will give you the bad news first: *If you have higher body fat, you burn fewer calories.* Those who start with a higher body fat percentage actually have to do *more* to get the same metabolic effect. Yes, a sluggish metabolism causes you to be even more sluggish (efficient), even though you may be moving more weight; you are burning fewer calories with the activity due to your higher proportion of insulin-resistant body fat, compared to insulin-sensitive muscle.

Now for the good news: *As body fat decreases and your fitness condition improves, your activities have a greater metabolic effect—meaning, you'll burn more calories.* Notice again that it's not about weight loss; your success relies upon lean muscle gain with a corresponding fat loss. Every percentage point of body fat lost makes your body more metabolically active. Compared to getting there, it is easy to maintain your leaner, healthier, more-insulin-sensitive body.

Remember to measure your progress without the scale. Your Blood Code will change with your effort, but forget what you've read about "calories burned during exercise." The effect of exercise is not measured by the spinning of a pedal on an exercise bike. Exercise machines and exercise charts painstakingly try to relate activities to calories burned.

The StairMaster may display 250 calories burned in 20 minutes, but that's not what has happened inside of you.

Myth #3: The layer of body fat on top of our core muscles does not respond to this kind of spot reduction. There is no need to focus on a single body part; again, the best exercise strategy is to engage more muscle groups than required for a given activity. Learn to engage your core with everything you do: a pull-back while on one leg, or a push-up with the added instability of an exercise ball. To get rid of your abdominal body fat, as I have said before in this book, you will need to lower insulin. The steps you have read about thus far will help you toward a leaner abdomen, not an "ab machine" advertised in a fitness magazine.

Myth #4: We have all been told over the years that stretching helps to prevent injury, and hot-room yoga took this myth to the next level. Stretching disengages some of the ability for a muscle to engage, or "fire," and has been shown to reduce athletic performance if done before the activity.[17] Remember: The goal is to engage *more* muscle fibers, not less. In truth, some stretching is helpful to some people, but most people have muscles that err on the side of flaccid—too much sitting, and not enough strenuous activity. Active engagement of your muscles throughout their range of motion is more important than a stretching routine. Deep lunge walking or any exercise that engages muscles throughout their full range of motion, *with resistance,* provides better results than static stretching.[18] This kind of dynamic strength training gives you the effect that you want from a stretch, and offers the metabolic reward of strength and better overall condition.

Step Six: Ensure Nutritional Support

Efficiency is doing things right; effectiveness is doing the right things.
—Peter Drucker, acclaimed management scholar

You will likely need additional nutrients beyond what a modern diet can provide to ensure that you have the healthiest function and best disease prevention. Over the past twenty years, I have worked in the supplement industry as a technical director, clinical consultant, lecturer, and author of medical research reviews for physicians and pharmacists. You might expect that with this experience, I would write about the latest and greatest herbs and nutrients that correct your health and metabolism. But, a bit of clinical and scientific skepticism can go a long way.

In the introduction I said, "Beware of any wellness plan that puts a pill ahead of dietary and fitness guidance." This is true. Nutritional supplements may be along for the ride on your health journey, but they're in the backseat. Supplemental nutrients serve to help you prevent the subtle deficiencies that might block your metabolism from properly responding to changes in your exercise and diet. The goal is to help you find a foundation to build upon; the house is your dietary and fitness lifestyle.

Therefore, I have distilled the bare essentials for a nutritional plan that will ensure that you are not deficient in the vitamins and minerals that support your health and metabolism. Here, in Step Six, there is no mega-dose, no over-glorified or unnecessary items.

> We all have to avoid being drawn into the hype of "miracle nutrient" headlines.
> These unrealistic claims disrupt our ability to see supplemental nutrients as an adjunctive piece of our wellness habits.

Nutrients and Your Metabolism

Nutrient Deficiencies Associated with Insulin Resistance

If your Blood Code displays insulin resistance, your cells likely have a nutritional deficiency or insufficiency that contributes to your compromised insulin response.[1] The primary nutrients that facilitate your healthy insulin response are *magnesium, vitamin D,* and *chromium.* The omega-3 essential fats found in fish oils have some powerful anti-inflammatory benefits, and can help to improve the TG:HDL ratio. Research on dietary fiber confirms that fibrous foods help to reduce the sugar load of a meal. Soluble fiber from vegetables has the most benefit of all, with over-the-counter fiber supplements not showing any significant benefit. Stick with food on this one.

You may experience nutrient deficiencies or insufficiencies that result in other non-insulin metabolic problems. The thyroid gland and thyroid hormone activation enzymes are made from the minerals iodine and selenium, and require zinc to work correctly. Your goal in The Blood Code Nutritional Plan is to avoid deficiency. When deficiency is no longer a factor, you can expect an optimal metabolic response from the important dietary and fitness steps that are to become your life habits.

What to Look For in a Vitamin/Mineral Combination

There is a marketing trend toward "whole foods" supplements. Most of these products include standard nutrients, with a "whole foods complex" added to the tablet or capsule contents. Your health is not served by taking a tablet with a two-year shelf life that contains an extra 50 mg of dried broccoli extract. Eat your broccoli and kale; the fresh or frozen vegetables deliver thousands of times more nutritional value than any pill. In fact, at a commonly used amount of 50 mg of vegetable extract, it would take you several *years* of taking the supplement to reach the equivalent of one 6-ounce serving of steamed broccoli. Use a nutritional supplement, from a reputable company, that provides mineral and vitamin nutrients in a well-balanced rational formula. Look for "whole foods" at your farmers' market and in the produce section, not on the supplement shelves.

Many professional-label supplement companies avoid the hype of over-the-counter market trends. If you work with a health-care provider who is well versed in nutritional evaluation and the nutritional companies available, you might want to go with their advice. You can also get more advice and up-to-date nutritional information by signing up for our newsletter at TheBloodCode.com.

Quality, Safety, and Reliability

I have consulted and worked for many nutritional and herbal supplement companies in the past twenty-five years. I have toured through dozens of facilities to view the steps they take for ingredient quality, safety, and verification. Prior to 2007, the FDA did not proactively police the manufacturing practices of nutritional supplement companies, and I saw the difference between companies that voluntarily met the higher-quality criteria and those that did not. There is no place in this industry for hidden and secretive practices. Here is what to avoid:

- **Proprietary blends:** I avoid using products that have "proprietary blends" of ingredients. When I call a company to get the actual amount of each ingredient that is listed, I want actual numbers—not to be told that it's a trade secret. Hogwash. These are supplements that I am asked to recommend to a person for their health, so full disclosure is imperative.

- **No manufacturer accountability:** As a health-care provider, I want to be able to talk to the actual manufacturer of any supplement product. The vast majority of multi-level marketed (MLM) products and direct-marketed items are labeled products from a different manufacturer. The manufacturer is kept secret. When I go to the supermarket I appreciate seeing which apple is from Washington and which is from Chile. Food and clothing retailers have responded to the public demand for source accountability; it's time for the supplement industry to follow suit.

- **Excessive hype:** The industry-allowed label claims border on the absurd. They are used to steer a buyer toward the product, not to provide meaningful information. You must find your information somewhere other than a label claim.

- **Imbalanced formulas:** Some individual nutrients are cheaper than others. Poorly designed, cheap nutrient combinations use an insignificant amount of the more-expensive nutrients and higher amounts of the cheaper ones. Nutrient combinations should be intelligently and rationally designed to provide a balance of the essential nutrients that provide what *you* are likely to need.

If you would like to compare the balance of nutrients in your current supplements, check the ingredients list at TheBloodCode.com for TBC Metabolic Support and TBC Metabolic Recovery. They contain equal parts magnesium-calcium, with a moderate vitamin and mineral content, and a high-potency fish oil capsule with 1,000 IU of added vitamin D. Meaningful doses of Coenzyme Q10 and alpha-lipoic acid are in the Recovery formula.

Why a Multiple Formula Is Better than Single Nutrients

Our bodies have evolved through eating foods that contain many nutrients that work synergistically. If you have a slight deficiency in one, there is likely a deficiency in other related nutrients. Certain nutrients are required for your metabolism, and if deficient, even by a small amount, complications and illness can result both quickly and over time.

A quick review of studies during the past few years in diabetes care reveals the importance of obtaining a complex of nutrients such as that found in a balanced multiple daily formula:

1. Vitamins C and E, zinc, and magnesium can prevent kidney damage in type 2 diabetics.[3]
2. Blood pressure reduces in diabetics when they take a multiple vitamin.[4]
3. Vitamins C and E, magnesium, and zinc are all associated with improvements in lipid panels, like increasing HDL-C.[81]
4. Vitamin D deficiency is associated with the onset of insulin resistance and diabetes.[5]

The body of research related to insulin resistance implies that there are subtle deficiencies that can trigger and complicate insulin resistance, and when these are corrected, outcomes improve. I cringe when a media headline claims "Vitamin D reverses diabetes." This claim is only going to generate a rebuttal, such as "Vitamin D fails to deliver on it's promise." This conflict is due to irrational, but profitable, sensationalism. Vitamin D deficiency is related to the insulin resistance of diabetes, and if uncorrected, diabetes is more difficult to reverse. But if you do noth-ing but pop a vitamin D pill, you will *not* reverse your diabetes, despite the wild claim. Nutritional guidance should not be sensational; instead, it should provide rational recommendations that support your health, performance, and disease prevention.

Nutrients with the Strongest Effect on Your Metabolism

Magnesium
USRDA= 300–350 mg
Blood Code Supplemental Range = 200–400 mg

Note: Above 400 mg, some people experience a loose bowel movement. Find your best tolerable dose.

In your body, magnesium is distributed quite evenly: approximately half in the bone, and half in the muscle and other soft tissues. Less than 1 percent is in your blood; thus, the blood test for magnesium is of little clinical use except in extreme hospital situations. Studies estimate that 75 percent of Americans do not meet the recommended dietary allowance of magnesium.[6] Magnesium deficiency is impli-cated, both cause and effect, in type 2 diabetes, metabolic syndrome, high blood pressure, cardiovascular disease, and inflammation. Magnesium is aptly included first in the list of clinically vital nutrients for your metabolism.[7]

Along with glucose and amino acids, magnesium is carried into your cells via the "insulin pump." Once your body is insulin-resistant, glucose and amino acids don't get taken into cells as readily, and neither does magnesium. *Resultant low intracellular magnesium causes condi-tions such as muscle pains, restless leg syndrome, insomnia, migraines, and high blood pressure.*[8] These conditions respond exceedingly well to extra magnesium supplementation. The going hypothesis is that as you develop insulin resistance, you become essentially magnesium-resistant. Given that most people take in less magnesium than the RDA indicates, magnesium supplementation is especially important if you have insulin resistance. Older people who have chronic insulin resistance are usually low in magnesium.[9]

Did you get that? As you age, you tend to be both low in, and resistant to, magnesium. A very well-designed study has proven that low brain magnesium is strongly associated with dementia; this is likely a reason why insulin resistance and Alzheimer's disease are linked. The same study showed that the healthier goal of *insulin sensitivity* was associated with higher and more-protective brain-cell magnesium levels.[10]

If high blood pressure develops in an adult for no obvious reason, assume magnesium deficiency and assess for insulin resistance.[11]

Most over-the-counter mineral supplements have an excessive amount of calcium, which might produce a relative magnesium deficiency. A "relative deficiency" occurs if you take an excess of one nutrient without the balance of other required nutrients. The relative imbalance can be as much of a problem as an overt nutritional deficiency. Magnesium and calcium should be supplemented near a 1:1 ratio. *Do not take high doses of straight calcium; anything over 500 to 600 milligrams per day is too much.*[12]

The best dietary sources of magnesium are cooked, dark leafy greens, broth from bones and connective tissues (like chicken bones), sunflower/pumpkin/ sesame seeds, legumes, and fish. (Dairy has high calcium, but almost no magnesium.)

Your daily supplement routine should deliver at least 200 mg of magnesium. If you take too much magnesium, you can experience a loose stool;

this can occur at higher doses in some people. Others might tolerate extra magnesium to help address symptoms of leg cramps and constipation.

Chromium
USRDA: Men = 30–35 mcg, Women = 20–30 mcg
Blood Code Supplemental Range = 50–100 mcg

Symptoms of chromium deficiency include severe insulin resistance, with high cholesterol and high glucose. Therefore, it makes sense that adding chromium might correct such a condition—but read on. The need for chromium is quite small; it is referred to as a *micro*nutrient due to the microgram dosage required. Chromium is found in stainless steel and most families of foods; therefore, true deficiency is extremely rare. Like many other micronutrients, such as selenium and manganese, toxicity can occur at only ten times the therapeutic dose, so high doses come with risks.

High-dose chromium supplementation was touted as a cure for obesity and diabetes for many years, and some of that hype remains in the air. However, more-comprehensive studies have failed to show any blood sugar improvements or weight loss with high-dose (>200 mcg) chromium supplementation.[13] A review of all placebo-controlled studies fails to reveal glucose improvement or heart disease risk reduction.[14]

So why is chromium in every diabetes and blood sugar protocol on the market? Because, inarguably, studies continue to show that if you are *deficient* in chromium, you are at high risk of insulin resistance and associated heart disease.[15] Your daily supplement should ensure that there is no chance of deficiency of this nutrient, without getting caught by the faddish excessive intake of supplemental chromium. Daily supplemental intake of 50 to 100 mcg is adequate, even if you have insulin resistance and elevated blood sugars.

Vitamin D
USRDA: Men and women, 600–800 IU
Blood Code Supplemental Range = 1,000–1,500 IU

Note: Your body can uniquely produce this vitamin when your skin is exposed to UVB rays from sunlight, but anything that blocks UVB, like sunblock lotion and glass windows, also blocks your body's ability to make vitamin D.

Experimental data have shown that vitamin D improves insulin resistance, exerts anti-inflammatory actions, and is important for glucose-induced insulin secretion. The link between low vitamin D in the bloodstream and stroke, heart attack, and high blood pressure is remarkably well-established.[16][17] Low blood vitamin D is also associated with countless other conditions, like cancers and autoimmune disease. The strong association between low vitamin D and the development of insulin resistance and type 2 diabetes is crystal clear.[18]

Despite all this associative data, numerous studies reveal a failure to "cure" insulin resistance with short-term use of high-dose supplemental vitamin D. Blood vitamin D levels are lower when people are insulin-resistant, and, for some reason, are higher in those without insulin resistance; it's not exactly cause and effect. Here again, you can appreciate the importance of implementing the right dietary and fitness steps for your Blood Code; mere vitamin D supplementation is not a magic bullet.[19]

Like chromium above, it is important that you avoid any chance of vitamin D deficiency. Your daily supplemental vitamin D intake should be between 1,000 and 1,500 IU. If you had low vitamin D on your Blood Code Discovery Panel, ensure a baseline recommended dose of vitamin D, and you should notice that your vitamin D level continues to improve as you become more insulin-sensitive. Your health-care provider might have good reason to use doses of vitamin D greater than 1,500 IU per day, but this should not be routine for everyone.

Vitamin K
USRDA: 90–120 mcg
Blood Code Optimal Dietary Intake: 300–600 mcg/day

Why food is the only way on this one: Studies indicate that additional vitamin K helps to improve insulin sensitivity, and while the USRDA is around 100 mcg, these studies used 500 mcg doses to improve heart health.[20] Vitamin K is a unique family of fat-soluble vitamins. Vitamin K1 is found in high amounts in dark, leafy green vegetables. When animals eat the K1 rich leafy greens, they produce higher levels of K2 in the fatty parts of their milk, meat, and eggs. Grains have no substantial vitamin K, so for humans and livestock, a grain-based diet harmfully restricts nutritional vitamin K intake. A diet rich in dark green vegetables along with dietary fats from grass-fed and pastured animals provides you with both vitamins K1 and K2, respectively.

Many physicians are nervous about people using supplemental vitamin K due to an interaction with frequently prescribed blood thinners, like Coumadin, even though a typical daily vitamin contains a paltry 50 mcg or less of vitamin K. Vitamin K1–rich dark leafy greens are incredibly nutrient-dense and disease-protective, and shouldn't be restricted. A cardiologist should not ask people to restrict these disease-protective foods. Instead, people should be asked to eat a very consistent amount of dark leafy greens, like 1/4 to 1/2 cup serving each day of some cooked dark leafy greens. If intake remains consistent, a blood thinner can be adjusted readily to accommodate a consistent dietary habit.

Most supplemental nutrient formulas, including The Metabolic Support Pack used at The Blood Code–Maine, contains no added vitamin K; *food sources of this vitamin need to be emphasized in your diet!* A small serving of 1/2 cup of cooked kale has over 500 mcg of vitamin K; additionally, it contains over 10,000 mcg of the wildly protective phytonutrients lutein and zeaxanthin. Five hundred mcg was the amount of vitamin K1 used in a study in diabetes care, which led to significant improvement in insulin resistance.[21]

> If my charge is to provide you with dietary and nutritional advice for your greatest health and disease prevention, then I must coach you toward a serving of dark green vegetables every day.
> —Dr. Richard Maurer

Fish Oils
Blood Code Supplemental Range: 1,000 mg of combined EPA and DHA
Equivalent to that found in about 3 ounces of cold-water fish

The active components of fish oil are the EPA and DHA fractions, long-chain omega-3 fatty acids. These two essential fats appear to powerfully decrease inflammation and atherogenic lipids, strongly and independently reducing heart disease risk. But fish oil does not likely improve insulin sensitivity and blood glucose control. The active omega-3 fatty acids improve several risk-associated components of the lipid panel; triglyceride decreases and LDL particle size increases. Without question, omega-3 rich fish oil has been shown to lower blood pressure and reduce inflammation.[22] With all this wonderful protective benefit at your door, more is better, right?

Rational readers should now realize that while some is good, more is *not* better. Studies using >3 to 6 grams of purified fish oils per day have displayed that insulin resistance markers actually worsen. The heart disease risks associated with lipid abnormalities can be reduced with a modest amount of fish oil, from quality fish, eggs, and meats from grass-fed beef and lamb. Your fish oil supplementation does not need to contain greater than 1,000 mcg of EPA and DHA.

Micro-Minerals for Thyroid Metabolism

Micro-minerals are those essential minerals *other than* calcium and magnesium. As the name implies, your need for these minerals is very small. For reference, a grain of sand weighs more than 10 micrograms, so a full complement of micro-minerals should be found in a properly balanced multiple vitamin-mineral supplement. Several micro-minerals are important regulators of your thyroid gland and thyroid activity. Your goal is to ensure that you are not deficient in these important building blocks for your metabolism.

Iodine: Blood Code Daily Intake Goal = 100–300 mcg/day

Iodine is the building block of the thyroid hormone. As home kitchens and food preparation move away from iodized salt toward more-natural sea salt, a little dose of iodine in a multiple is a wise idea. If you are vulnerable to hypothyroid, inadequate intake of iodine in your diet can affect your metabolism and/or lower thyroid hormone production.

Your daily supplement of iodine should be 50 to 100 mcg/day. Amounts higher than 300 mcg can be harmful and suppress peripheral thyroid activity.[23]

Food sources of iodine include saltwater fish and shellfish, which contain close to 100 mcg of iodine; a single ounce of dry seaweed can contain 200 to 400 mcg of iodine. Dairy products, such as plain whole yogurt, contain 50 to 75 mcg per serving.

Selenium: Blood Code Daily Intake Goal = 50–100 mcg/day

Just like iodine is the building block of your thyroid hormone, selenium is the building block of the enzyme that activates your thyroid hormone. And again, if you are vulnerable to hypothyroid, i.e., with an elevated TPO antibody, a little selenium deficiency can make your thyroid problem much worse.[24] It does not take a lot of selenium to prevent deficiency, and the small amount in a proper multiple vitamin-mineral is an adequate safeguard for the days when dietary selenium is inadequate.

Your daily supplement of selenium should be 50 to 100 mcg.

Food sources of selenium include nuts, seeds, fish, poultry, and beef, all of which contain 25 to 50 mcg per serving. Brazil nuts have a whopping 500 mcg per handful.

Zinc: Blood Code Daily Intake Goal = 10–20 mg/day

Zinc is one of the most widely required nutrients in your body. Both insulin and thyroid hormone actively rely on adequate zinc in your daily diet. Small amounts go a long way. Typical zinc supplements in their own capsule contain an excessive 50 mg; this amount can result in anemia over time, and should be avoided.

Your daily supplement of zinc should be 5 to 10 mg, to ensure that you are not deficient.

Food sources of zinc include meats, poultry, and seafood, which contain 10 to 20 mg per serving. Oysters are the standout, with up to 200 mg in only 3 ounces.

Coenzyme Q10 / CoQ10 and Alpha-Lipoic Acid (ALA)

These two unique nutrients receive attention for type 2 diabetes, insulin resistance, and metabolism.

> **Coenzyme Q10 / CoQ10:** Coenzyme Q10 has another name, Ubiquinol, a reference to its ubiquitous presence in every cell throughout the body. The unfortunate popularity of "statin" medication for lowering blood cholesterol put CoQ10 on the map of research in the past decades because these medications problematically cause a drop in tissue CoQ10 levels. This biochemical result from cholesterol medications is likely behind the statin side effects of muscle pain, weakness, and fatigue. CoQ10 supplementation is more indicated for people with elevated lipids, elevated blood pressure, and elevated blood glucose.[25]

According to researchers, "CoQ10 supplementation may improve blood pressure and long-term glycemic control in subjects with type 2 diabetes."[26]

Due to drug interactions, you might require CoQ10. Medical prescribing manuals recommend supplemental CoQ10 for those on beta-blockers and statin medications.[27]

Athletes at peak condition can generate slightly more peak performance if they take CoQ10 along with intensive training. Okay, I realize this study was on absolute peak performance in athletes, which does not relate to most of us, but it reinforces a supportive role for CoQ10 with exercise.[28]

Food Sources of CoQ10: There is CoQ10 naturally in "muscular" meats; heart and tongue are uniquely rich in CoQ10, but are, not surprisingly, absent in most modern diets. Red meat and poultry typically provide all the CoQ10 in today's modern American diet, but it only adds up to about 5 mg daily. CoQ10 is absorbed similarly from food and supplements.[29] There are no vegetarian sources of CoQ10.

Blood Code Supplemental Range for CoQ10 = 50–100 mg: Research was often for four- to twelve-week periods, and used 100 to 200 mg per day. A dose of 200 mg per day resulted in a threefold increase in blood CoQ10 levels in study subjects in a short period of time. A long-term daily supplement of 50 to 100 mg will raise blood levels adequately, and is recommended if you have high blood glucose, high blood pressure, and/or high blood lipids.

Alpha-Lipoic Acid (ALA): For many years, the antioxidant and protective effect of supplemental alpha-lipoic acid on people with diabetic nerve damage was well established. Now, numerous studies over the past ten years have confirmed that there is a clinical indication for alpha-lipoic acid for people with insulin resistance. Many of these studies were short-term and utilized much higher-dose alpha-lipoic acid than you would take on a daily basis, but the results were impressive.

ALA helps you move toward insulin sensitivity: Relatively small studies on people with type 2 diabetes displayed that very high-dose supplementation can recover insulin sensitivity similar to that of nondiabetic controls.[30][31]

ALA works synergistically with exercise: People who express insulin resistance experience greater correction of their insulin problem if they take supplemental alpha-lipoic acid in conjunction with exercise. When exercise and ALA are used together, the correction of insulin resistance is greater than either therapy on its own. *This again reinforces the idea that supplements are supportive; they are not replacements for good diet and fitness habits!*[32]

ALA works better on those with already-good glycemic control: This small but recent study simply compared a short course of alpha-lipoic acid treatment on type 2 diabetes. It found that those with better control of their blood sugar had a better response to ALA compared to those that took the nutrient but did not have as good glucose control. Sound familiar? Nutrients can be adjunctive and supportive, not some stand-alone miracle.[33]

Food Sources of ALA: Vegetables have only trace amounts of alpha-lipoic acid, found in beets, broccoli, Brussels sprouts, carrots, tomatoes, and yams. Red meat, and particularly organ meat, is an excellent source of ALA, albeit, still lower than supplementation provides.

Blood Code Supplemental Range for ALA = 50–100 mg/day: While many of the short-term studies used up to 600 mg or more, these studies were three weeks to three months long. Long-term daily supplementation can be as low as 50 mg per day.

Herbal Therapies

Herbal Supplements and Your Blood Sugar Metabolism—Why and Why Not?

Daily herbal supplements are not part of your Blood Code program, unless you consider the potent herbal extracts of tea and coffee, used daily by billions of us. I have never seen any herbal extract work even one-tenth as well as a little bit of exercise or appropriate diet change. There *is* evidence that herbal treatments can have an effect on blood sugars; I will review the ones that have the strongest evidence base here, and describe why I do not include them in your supplemental recommendations.

Berberine extract: If you have perused the online recommendation for the symptom of high blood sugar, you have probably come across berberine sulphate. Berberine is the extracted alkaloid from the Oregon grape / barberry family of plants. It has potent hypoglycemic effects, and beginning around 1990, has been confirmed as a useful substance to help improve blood sugars, while lowering insulin and central body fat distribution. It has won a reputation for being "like metformin," the common first-line drug for type 2 diabetes.[34]

The mechanism for berberine extract is very unclear. For decades it has been a well-researched herbal treatment for intestinal infections, like Giardia, but it came with the warning to avoid long-term use due to the potential undesirable and antimicrobial effect in the gut. Significant gastrointestinal side effects are well documented with berberine extract studies.

The gastrointestinal side effect of malabsorption is likely the primary reason why berberine lowers post-meal blood sugar; the herb is not absorbed, and acts within the gut to cause malabsorption of glucose and potentially other important nutrients.[35] In the type 2 diabetes study, over 30 percent of the subjects that took berberine sulphate had side effects including digestive distress, nausea, and diarrhea.[36] The frequency of GI side effects reinforces how the herb likely works to reduce blood sugars—by creating malabsorption, so the meal nutrients go right through.[37] It is better for you to put less carbohydrate in your mouth than to take a drug that causes gastrointestinal irritation and interferes with nutrient absorption. This extract is available over the counter, but at this time, I don't recommend pursuing this herbal extract as therapy for hyperglycemia or type 2 diabetes.

Cinnamon: More than a few studies have negated the initial hype about using cinnamon to reduce blood sugar. While the polyphenolic extract of cinnamon (*Cinnamomum cassia*) does show some minor effects that could help people with type 2 diabetes, the effect is so small that well-designed studies fail to confirm any benefit.[38] But is there harm in using a teaspoon of cinnamon in your foods on a daily basis? None at all; enjoy.

Gymnema sylvestre: An herbal extract from the leaf of a traditional Ayurvedic plant, this is in nearly every "diabetic support formula" on the market. I used to use this myself, and my lower blood sugar results were undeniable. But how does it work? Your body releases *more* insulin.[39] Since this is the very problem you are trying to avoid, and since other drugs that raise insulin are associated with long-term complications and death in type 2 diabetics, this herbal extract is not part of a long-term plan in the Blood Code.

American ginseng (aka, *Panax quinquefolius*): Researchers have shown that high doses of Panax ginseng extract, when used before a high-carb meal, reduce blood sugar in the hours after the meal. While this sounds interesting, it is a similar effect found with alcohol. The sugar is still ingested, so if it isn't in the bloodstream right away, where is it? Did it quickly get turned into fat or glycogen? Is the glucose now in your liver? When nondiabetics took Panax ginseng well before a meal, their blood sugars dropped substantially. It does appear now that the primary mechanism of Panax ginseng to lower blood sugar is to raise insulin, which in turn causes more fat production. Remember: Insulin resistance and high insulin, not high blood sugar, is the problem behind heart disease and diabetes. Panax ginseng is a very interesting herb with many diverse effects, but it shouldn't be part of a long-term plan if you need to control your blood sugars.[40][41]

My supplement routine . . .

I do best when I take a low dose of a well-balanced multiple. Extra calcium and magnesium help my muscles to relax. If I am on my one-coffee-per-day habit, I need extra cal-mag to prevent my muscles from tightening at night and with exercise. My skin is better with a little fish oil and vitamin D. Alas, I am admittedly bad at remembering to take my vitamins individually, even though I feel better with them. For convenience, I usually take the multi-dose pack developed through The Blood Code (with me in mind) with breakfast or dinner, whichever I can remember. –Dr. Richard Maurer

You now understand nutritional supplementation for what it is—a supplement to your diet and lifestyle habits. For years I have seen new patients arrive at my office with only five to six hours of sleep per night, complaining of fatigue. They usually have a long list of nutrients and herbs, recommended by well-meaning practitioners, and they can't understand why "the treatments aren't working."

Lifestyle changes need to be first and foremost. Certain medications and underlying medical conditions raise the need for certain nutrients and herbal therapies, and you will be best served if you see a health-care provider with knowledge and understanding of natural therapies. There are other stresses and lifestyle factors that might need to be addressed and assessed, which we will review in the next chapter.

Lifestyle Habits that Support Your Steps: Alcohol, Sleep, and Stress

Alcohol, sleep patterns, and stress management all play a role in your metabolism. Good habits have you covered. But what constitutes "good"? Medical research has yet to reach a consensus on exactly what constitutes moderate alcohol intake, although recommendations have settled at one drink per day for women, and two for men. As regards the appropriate amount of sleep per night, how do you know what is enough? And just what is good stress management? Let's review the answers with an eye toward your metabolic health and longevity.

Alcohol and Your Metabolism

Simply put, alcohol deranges your carbohydrate metabolism.

That sounds bad, doesn't it? But the verbiage is apt. Alcohol reduces the amount of fat the body burns for energy. As your body breaks down alcohol, the compounds formed (acetate) affect both your pancreas and liver, and replace and prevent your normal fat-burning metabolism. Alcohol causes your liver to hold on to stored sugar and fat dearly; you become a fat-storage machine *and* a miser.

If you're trying to improve your athletic performance, alcohol inhibits the release of glycogen and fats, which are needed to sustain a physical activity. Athletic performance takes a nosedive with alcohol around.

If you're trying to lower your body fat, alcohol triggers the storage of fats and carbohydrates. Like the athlete's dilemma, fat will not be burned with alcohol around, and furthermore, additional fat will be deposited.

If you have high insulin or fatty liver, alcohol is a dangerous friend. The damaging effects from fatty liver disease and the stress to the pancreas result in morbid outcomes.

If blood sugar irregularities are an issue, alcohol is again a villain. Alcohol, in fact, lowers blood sugar levels when consumed. This occurs because the resultant acetate prevents your liver from releasing the stored glycogen and fat as blood sugar.

Carbs in Alcohol: The Much Smaller Half of the Story

The carb count of alcohol is misleading, as just noted. It's alcohol's problematic effect on your metabolism which is important to you, not just the calorie count. Whether an alcoholic drink claims to be low-carb or not, the alcohol content of a "drink" is the same. A serving of alcohol, or "a drink," is defined as follows:

> Beer: 12 ounces
> Wine: 5 ounces
> Distilled liquor: 1.5 ounces

Each serving of alcohol has between 12 to 14 grams of alcohol. This adds up to about 100 calories. Calorically, the alcohol part of a drink is counted like a fat—thus, the high caloric value of alcoholic drinks—but metabolically, in your body, it does not behave at all like dietary fat.

The residual carbohydrate content varies from drink to drink, but again, the alcohol content of each drink below is the same, so the "derangement" of your metabolism is the same due to the alcohol.

Obviously, the worst drinks for you are the ones with alcohol *and* sugars, such as a liquor with soda. Yes, there are things out there called "alcopops"—alcohol and soda combined. It goes without saying that you should avoid these!

The residual carbohydrate content in "a drink" is a small part of the total calories.

> Regular beer: 12 to 14 grams carb
> Light beer: 4 to 6 grams carb
> Wine: 2 to 4 grams carb
> Distilled liquor: 0 grams carb

The carb content from alcoholic beverages is, of course, "empty carbohydrates"; there is no nutritional value. You should count the carb grams according to your Blood Code carbohydrate ranges, always keeping in mind that the grams of alcohol require respect. You need to understand what your body will do with the complex set of metabolic storage effects from alcoholic drinks.

How much alcohol is too much? The issue of alcohol is a complicated one, and requires more than simply deeming your consumption good or bad. Alcohol tolerance is about *you!*

If you have a fasting insulin above 8, or if you have a TG above 100, you should restrict your alcohol to less than one drink per day on average. Your body has proven that it is really good at fat storage, and alcohol will act as a turbo boost to this process.

If your skin-fold caliper measurement is highest on your hip, you should restrict alcohol as much as possible. Alcohol is an empty sugar that effectively promotes fat storage, so if it were any other food, like a chocolate-frosted cookie, it would be on the *avoid* list.

In my opinion . . .

How much alcohol is just right can't be answered en masse. Large-scale studies show some heart disease protection with low to moderate alcohol intake, presumably due to its ability to lower blood pressure, but cancer studies are not so forgiving. Medically, there is nothing beneficial that happens after two drinks, and for many people, benefits stop closer to one drink.

All that said, in small amounts of one drink or less, I think that the fat-storing metabolic effect of alcohol is probably manageable for most of you. But you should watch your Blood Code Panel results and assess your fat-storage and fat-burning capacity. If you are not getting the results that you want or expect with your current dietary and fitness habits, your alcohol intake may be an area that needs attention and reduction.

Sleep and Your Metabolism

A study in 2007 showed that there were profound metabolic changes occurring in adults who were sleep-deprived, even during a single night. But after this study, the question still remains: How much sleep is enough?[1]

A comparative study done in 2010 looked at the effect of different amounts of sleep on dieters. Subjects who slept for five and a half hours retained more body fat than those who slept for eight and a half hours, even though both groups lost the same amount of weight. This means that if you lose weight, you will lose more muscle if you are under-slept. Furthermore, the people in the sleep-deprived group felt less satisfied overall, and hungrier. It was not a surprise to the researchers that this group had higher levels of the hormone *ghrelin,* a hormone that drives the feeling for hunger and cravings. *You cannot maintain healthy weight and metabolism while remaining under-slept.*[2]

Granted, like most studies, statistical significance is found at the extremes; five and a half versus eight and a half hours' sleep is a big difference. When researchers compare seven versus eight hours of sleep, the difference is minor, but less than six hours compared to more than eight—bingo!

My sleep habits: In a world of productivity and electronic distractions, we all need to be reminded of the critical value of sleep. I personally try to average about seven and a half to eight hours per night, and more if I am training; fewer hours remains the exception.
-Dr. Richard Maurer

Sleep and Metabolism in Kids

A study in the *Journal of Pediatrics* in February 2011 found erratic sleep patterns were associated with metabolic syndrome findings . . . in four- to ten-year-olds! True, the findings don't necessarily prove cause and effect, but the feast-or-famine practice of sleep deprivation on school nights and "sleeping in" on weekends was associated with obesity and the beginning of insulin resistance.

This study stands out for many reasons: First is the age of the participants, four- to ten-year-olds. It is fully appropriate to assess The Blood Code before adulthood. Second are the blood tests that were ordered. The researchers performed insulin, glucose, and lipid panels on these kids. In the thousands of children I have seen in my office, I have yet to observe many physicians who ordered the simple and revealing blood tests of insulin and lipids for a child. Step One of The Blood Code teaches you how to unlock these answers for yourself. Third is the confirmation that lack of sleep results in muscle loss rather than fat loss, again showing that the scale misleads you; skin-fold calipers are a superior measurement of metabolic health. So while diet and exercise get all the attention, adequate and regular sleep habits also play an important role in your metabolism from an early age.[3]

Stress and Your Blood Code

Things do not change; we change.
—Henry David Thoreau

Whenever people try to describe the stress in their life, they invariably talk about the things that are happening around them. How you perceive and respond to events in your life is what creates more or less of a stress response. Most modern-day stresses are not short-term, physical, fight-or-flight type events. Consecutive work deadlines, unavoidable daily stresses, chronic illness, family tensions—the list includes events that do not end tomorrow. Studies show that chronic stress can put you on the fast track toward weight gain and metabolic syndrome if high dietary carbohydrate triggers exist too.[4] You must have a plan to help control the adverse effects of chronic stress.

I am aware that plenty of previously released books have detailed the impact of chronic stress on your health, and perhaps that's why this section sits so deep in this book. But I'd like to throw in my emphasis here: *Unresolved stress can actually precipitate insulin resistance, and all the heart disease risks that go with it.*[5] Stress management should not be seen as a "sidebar" to your other life activities.

The good news? It's really easy. Like exercise, a little bit might actually go a long way. Studies have shown a dramatic reduction in stress hormones just by taking a few relaxed, deep breaths. I'm not talking about a one-hour meditation class here; the evidence supports taking a few deep breaths every hour; yeah, just a few!

Here are three research-proven ways to reduce the harmful effects of chronic stress:

1) Deep breathing, *even just a few breaths,* results in significant hormonal improvement. Stress hormones in your body release instantaneously, but they clear quickly as well, given the right stimulus, such as a deep, relaxed breath.

2) Physical contact with others, the opposite of social isolation, leads to instantaneous hormonal improvement.

3) Short naps, 20 minutes or less, can result in dramatic physical and mental benefits. Many people think a nap will slow them down, but if you keep it to 20 minutes or less, it will actually improve your metabolism.

This is a good time to mention caffeine . . .

Like alcohol, people try to pass moral judgment on coffee, but it is neither good nor bad. *Know thyself* is the real answer. Coffee is a digestive stimulant, so gastrointestinal irritation is a common side effect from coffee. Coffee and tea both contain caffeine; 12 ounces of drip coffee has about 200 mg, and tea has about 65 mg per tea bag. Therefore, they are both stimulants, coffee to a greater degree. You do not need a stimulant if you are sitting still at a desk; your muscles will tighten up. If you are going to exercise or be active, the caffeine is better tolerated. Like many drug effects, your body will build up a tolerance to caffeine if ingested daily. Athletes who use it for exercise performance will avoid it for weeks prior to an event, then drink it on race day for added muscular activity.

Be kind . . . to yourself!

Books such as Jean Fain's *The Self-Compassion Diet* and Kristin Neff's 2011 book, *Self-Compassion: Stop Beating Yourself Up and Leave Insecurity Behind,* make scientific arguments that guilt and self-critical emotions actually lower compliance, and are associated with poor eating and exercise habits. Dr. Neff states, "Self-compassion is really conducive to motivation." This will require practice if your first thoughts are about how fat you are, or how bad you are because you eat the wrong things. Science concurs that you need to start with a state of acceptance and mindfulness.

The knowledge and understanding you gain from your Blood Code provides you with an acceptable explanation of your current metabolism. And remember: Self-acceptance does not result in laziness; it's a firm stone from which to leap!

Digging Deeper: Confidence through Research

We must not be hampered by yesterday's myths in concentrating on today's needs.
—Harold S. Geneen, businessman, former CEO of ITT

You are becoming your own authority. If you display significant insulin resistance, you know that your body has a unique need for a low-carb and high-fat diet. There will always be low-fat advocates, and people who, despite the evidence, believe that cholesterol is bad. Period. You need to be free to make the unbiased dietary and fitness changes that meaningfully and effectively improve your own personal health.

In this section, I will offer a more research-oriented explanation behind four major Blood Code topics that patients have grappled with over the years.

1. The research related to low-fat versus lower-carb / high-fat diets
2. Cholesterol: the hype and the myths
3. The research behind using TG:HDL ratio, insulin, and insulin resistance as markers of true health and disease prevention
4. The medical mistake of merely treating the glucose in people with type 2 diabetes

The Low-Fat Diet Is Dead

Sorry to be so blunt, but there is no scientific basis to promote the health benefits of a low-fat diet. To resolve and reverse insulin resistance and cardiometabolic disease, fat is the one food that does not require insulin from your pancreas. Throughout this book, you have been instructed to include dietary fats in place of carbs to promote your healthiest metabolism; if this was surprising news for you, read on.

Back in 2003, a diet study actually did what few studies had ever done before: Rather than after-the-fact questionnaires, people were fed three daily meals at a restaurant, so exact meals could be prepared and supervised. The study compared the weight-loss effects of a low-carb, *high-fat* diet of 1,800 calories and a *low-fat,* high-carb diet of 1,500 calories. Not only did the low-carb / high-fat (Blood Code type) group lose more weight, they also reported feeling more satisfied. Even with fewer calories, the low-fat group fared worse for weight loss.[6] Critics of the study went so far as to say, "It doesn't make sense, does it? It violates the laws of thermodynamics."

Well, as far as this author knows, nothing has broken the second law of thermodynamics in our universe to date. Lead researcher Dr. Greene astutely responded, "I don't think for a minute that anything is violating the laws of thermodynamics. . . . There's no smoke and mirrors here."

Another criticism of this landmark study was the mythological belief that the high-fat diet would ultimately cause heart disease.

Enter the follow-up study. Between 2005 and 2007, a two-year study was designed to promote weight loss in an overweight population, but this time, heart disease risk factors would be monitored throughout the study (blood pressure, lipids, inflammation, and so on). Furthermore, the study had a third study group, the Mediterranean diet.

The Mediterranean and low-fat groups were advised to stay within caloric restrictions of 1,500 calories for women and 1,800 for men. This is significant caloric restriction for most people; therefore, dietitians met with the groups regularly for instruction and motivation. The low-carb /

high-fat group was not given caloric restrictions; *their quantity was "self-regulated."*

The higher-fat diet resulted in a more-favorable effect on blood lipid levels. The high-fat group added more dietary protein, cholesterol, and fats than the other groups, but had the most substantial TG:HDL improvements. After reading this book, you know why, right? The high-fat group had lower insulin throughout the study term.[7]

The effect of better self-regulation is no small finding here. People with the higher-fat and lower-carb intake naturally controlled their food intake better than the other groups. Since you don't all have calorie cops calling you monthly for motivation sessions, you need to find a diet that satisfies you for the rest of your life.

The low-fat group fared the worst again, despite the lowest caloric intake (200 calories less than the other groups). The low-fat diet led to the smallest amount of weight loss and the worst cardiac numbers compared to the Mediterranean and the high-fat diet. In a mark of poor sportsmanship, a popular low-fat advocate was quoted as saying, "I'm also very skeptical of the quality of data in this study. [The results are] physiologically impossible."

Here we go again: A medical authority claims that some law of physics must have been broken rather than admit that a statistically significant number of people are harmed by a low-fat diet.

Well-regarded dietary studies since 2008 continue to confirm the benefits of the reduced-carbohydrate Blood Code style diet.[8][9][10][11]

A meta-analysis study in Sweden was completed in October of 2013—and an overseeing committee member, Prof. Frederik Nystrom, summarized succinctly, "Our deep seated fear of fat is completely unfounded. You don't get fat from fatty foods, just as you don't get atherosclerosis from calcium or turn green from green vegetables." In contrast to the United States, where the processed food industry carries too much influence over health policy, Sweden chose to reject any low fat recommendations and instead encourage the intake of whole saturated fats to replace excess carbs.[12]

Cholesterol—The Hype and the Myth

You will notice that little attention is placed on total and LDL cholesterol in The Blood Code. That is because it's not an accurate or helpful indicator of your health and longevity.[13] A 2009 American Medical Association (AMA) publication stated that all physicians should be running blood tests such as insulin to identify those patients at risk for high blood pressure and heart disease.[14] Years have passed, and cholesterol still dominates the market and conversation, in large part due to the marketing of statin medications, the most financially lucrative drug class to have ever hit the market worldwide.

Statins, the drugs that lower cholesterol, have enjoyed nearly two decades' worth of publicity in which billions upon billions of dollars have been spent in advertising campaigns to convince you and your doctor that you will reduce your risk of heart attack and stroke if you take the medication. The fact is that only about 1 percent of high-risk people taking the drug will reduce their stroke or heart attack incidence. Women, and those over the age of seventy, don't even get the 1 percent reduction. And one more thing: Studies show that those who take the drug don't live longer, so apparently, they die more often from other stuff.[15]

I love science and the rational interpretation that must be exercised when evaluating research. The pharmaceutical industry has creatively packaged statistics into brochures and commercials, and they are really good at it. In my experience, when a drug goes generic, the industry spin stops, and some of the truth begins to come out. In the case of statins, Pfizer's blockbuster statin drug, Lipitor, went generic in January of 2012.

Here are some headlines from WebMD from the following six months:

February 28, 2012: FDA ADDS WARNINGS TO STATIN LABEL: DIABETES, MEMORY LOSS, HIGH BLOOD SUGARS by Reed Miller
June 11, 2012: STATINS LINKED TO FATIGUE IN RANDOMIZED STUDY by Sue Hughes

August 13, 2012: STATINS LINKED WITH DEVELOPMENT OF CATA-
RACTS by Michael O'Riordan
August 22, 2012: STATIN POTENCY LINKED WITH MUSCLE WEAK-
NESS by Nancy A. Melville
March 1, 2013: STATIN THERAPY AND THE RISK FOR DIABETES
AMONG ADULT WOMEN: DO THE BENEFITS OUTWEIGH THE RISK?
by Yunsheng Ma, et al.
June 5, 2013: STATINS LINKED WITH RISK OF MUSCULOSKELETAL
INJURY by Michael O'Riordan

Despite damaging side effects, statin-type cholesterol-lowering medication has been prescribed with abandon for two decades, and yet scientific evidence does not show any significant reduction in death rates for those using the drug for primary prevention of heart attack and stroke.[16]

Once you depart from the LDL cholesterol fixation, you can appreciate the other parts of your Blood Code that realistically signify your path to health and longevity: TG:HDL, insulin, HOMA-IR, and body fat distribution.

Your Triglyceride/HDL Ratio and Insulin Level

Your Triglyceride/HDL ratio and insulin level offer a lifelong metric for your health.

TG:HDL is one of the criteria for the diagnosis of metabolic syndrome, which was briefly known as Reaven's syndrome, named after Gerald Reaven, MD, of Stanford University. He and his colleagues around the world pioneered much of the early research on blood tests and body fat distribution that indicates cardiovascular risk.[17] TG:HDL is a strong marker of lifestyle factors—perhaps a reason it is ignored in most pharmaceutically oriented medical offices.

Your TG:HDL ratio offers a way to see whether you have a metabolism that naturally has cardiac protection (the lucky ones), or whether you need to earn it (like me). Let me explain the studies.

Three thousand people were categorized for known risk factors for heart attack and stroke: smoking, high blood pressure, or a sedentary lifestyle. In all of the categories, those with the higher TG:HDL ratios (>3) had the highest incidence of heart attacks and strokes, compared to those with the lowest ratio (<1.1), and the incidence of events was linear with the TG:HDL ratio.

In fact, the group that had the lower ratio and smoked cigarettes had no more cardiac events than nonsmokers. This particular finding entertained journalists, who concluded that "You can smoke if you have a low TG:HDL ratio." Remember, this study only looked at cardiovascular disease, not cancer, so I still advise restraint. Know your TG:HDL ratio, and keep yourself in the lower range, as close to 1 as possible.[18]

Triglyceride is not an adequate test on its own. As TG goes up, the fat and sugar is stored in the liver, making it less able to function properly. Therefore, the liver does not produce the healthful HDL. The medical journals refer to this condition as *diabetic atherogenic dyslipidemia*. Intimidating name, but as it implies, when these lipids get out of balance, atherosclerosis and heart disease follow; and likewise, your disease risk goes down with improvement in your TG:HDL.

Insulin and the HOMA-IR marks for disease risk and **your healthy life:** High insulin results in central obesity and high blood pressure. There is a strong link to heart attack and stroke with high insulin.[19] There is a strong link between elevated fasting insulin and breast cancer,[20] melanoma,[21] and colon cancer risk.[22] I could list more nondiabetic conditions associated with high insulin, but I have to stop somewhere, and this list already includes the top five causes of death in the U.S. I am stunned that health-care providers do not run a fasting insulin test routinely, and I am further convinced that it's time for you to get in the driver's seat of your own health and prevention and run these tests!

Insulin has so many mechanisms to raise heart disease risk, cancer risk, and trigger inflammation.

Insulin induces sodium retention at the kidney, causing excess fluid retention, which worsens inflammation and raises blood pressure.[23] Insulin, as you know, raises the TG, but it also decreases the size of the LDL particle, to a size more associated with atherosclerosis formation.[24] Insulin raises the levels of uric acid, causing high blood pressure and the condition called *gout*. Insulin can affect other hormones, as seen in the condition called *polycystic ovary syndrome* (PCOS), where women experience hormonal imbalance associated with high insulin.

High insulin is the driving force behind fat deposits in the liver, called *benign hepatic steatosis*. The word *benign* is a bit of a misnomer; while this cause of fatty liver is not a precursor to liver cancer or hepatitis, it is a recipe for heart disease.[25] Statistically, over 70 percent of adults with fatty liver are obese, but there are lean individuals with excess fat deposits "inside" their body.[26] [27]

Longevity is associated with people who have *lower insulin* levels and a low HOMA-IR that reflects insulin sensitivity.[28] This compelling research brings into question one of the greatest mistakes of pharmaceutical-based medical care: the treatment of type 2 diabetes with drugs that actually *raise* insulin.

The Foolish Mistake of Treating Glucose and Not Insulin Resistance

The medical establishment has failed when it comes to fighting "the war" on type 2 diabetes. First, there is no war, and even if there was, the enemy has been misidentified. The underlying condition that leads to type 2 diabetes is not obesity; it's not overeating; it's not laziness. *It is insulin resistance.* I think we can all understand that if you put drugs that raise insulin into someone to help lower their sugar, you will actually make the underlying problem—insulin resistance—worse.

In a large-scale study called the ACCORD trial, published in the *New England Journal of Medicine* in 2008, type 2 diabetics were divided into groups to compare more-aggressive combined drug therapy to lower blood glucose levels to as close to normal as possible (goal was <6). But the study did nothing to emphasize diet and exercise; researchers were instead going to use what most doctors use already, "polypharmacy"—many different drugs in each person as needed to lower sugars, like metformin, glipizide (one of many drugs that trigger more insulin secretion), and injectable insulin. The trial was planned for 5.6 years, but was discontinued after 3.5 years because the people on more-intensive drug protocols were dying far more rapidly than the controls, even though they had lower average blood sugars, measured by A1C. The lead author, Dr. Hertzel Gerstein, explained the incriminating findings: "We believe that some unidentified combination of factors tied to the overall medical strategy is likely at play."[29]

Overall medical strategy means that the entire concept of drugging the body into metabolic submission (lowering blood glucose was the only goal of therapy) kills more people than it cures. Glucose isn't the culprit; insulin resistance is the culprit. The people in the aggressively treated group took medications that raised their insulin levels (glipizide, insulin), thereby making their insulin resistance worse. Drug-induced high insulin, just like innate high insulin, causes fat gain, fluid retention, even more insulin resistance, and blood sugar irregularities. People in the ACCORD trial were not instructed to reduce their carbohydrate intake. I will again state an apparent truth: The medical-industrial-pharmaceutical system has no vested interest in advising *you* to prevent or reverse disease through lifestyle.

In a related news event in the *New York Times* (June 3, 2013), reporters covered the unusual move of the US FDA, which announced that it might retract its prior restrictions on the drug Avandia, a diabetes drug that raises insulin but increased the incidence of heart attacks. The article was not in the health section; it was in the business section.

The FDA decision was seen as a "huge victory for the drug maker, GlaxoSmithKline." Their huge victory is a colossal loss for all those people who look to their doctors for guidance toward "the best" therapy for type 2 diabetes.

In short, there is not a drug or miracle pill that helps you correct insulin resistance. And even though there are drugs to lower your sugar, you will have to accept a shorter and sicker life. If you have type 2 diabetes, you need to guide your own diet and lifestyle to reverse disease and restore your health.

How Your Blood Code Relates to Other Hormones in Your Body

I receive countless e-mails from supplement companies and sales reps who claim to have a product that will cure hormone imbalance. The products have evocative names like Corti-stim or Corti-calm or Lepti-slim. To better understand your underlying metabolism in the world of hormone hype, I will rationally describe the most popular hormones that are marketed for your metabolism. If these are new terms for you, just consider this section a basic introduction. These hormones are not critical to your success, just interesting players.

Leptin and Adiponectin

The past twenty years has been very exciting for metabolism geeks like myself. Until the early 1990s, fat tissue was considered passive tissue; it was just the "stuff in the way" of other tissues. Now fat tissue is understood as a dynamic endocrine organ of the body, a gland communicating with all the other parts of your endocrine system. In medical language, fat is not called *fat*; it rises to the name *adipose,* and the hormonal compounds that get released from adipose are called *adipocytokines.* There are two primary adipocytokines that your body releases throughout the day, leptin and adiponectin, and together, they signal numerous actions related to glucose and fat utilization and hunger.[30]

Leptin is only secreted by the fat cells, and its job is to turn off your hunger. The more fat cells you have, the higher your leptin. Sensibly, your body does not need more food if you already have so many fat cells, so hunger is shut off. In a perfect world, lean people have less leptin and therefore are hungrier, and obese people will have more leptin, less appetite, and eat less. Even in the short term, leptin levels drop if there has been a sudden drop in caloric intake, so hunger can be triggered. Why doesn't this system always work, then?

Enter *leptin resistance*. While the actions of leptin and adiponectin are still under investigation in the scientific community, it is clear that humans experience the same trends with leptin resistance and adiponectin resistance as with insulin resistance.[31] Chronically high levels of leptin will create the same "boy who cried wolf" scenario with leptin. Your brain will just stop listening to the message of leptin, and your appetite will never be turned off, even after a meal. What keeps your leptin chronically high? Living with a higher-than-normal body fat percentage and never adequately fasting. The subtle message of chronically elevated leptin can become background noise in your metabolic chorus, leaving you to ignore its simple message.

Snacks between meals and eating before bedtime are the best ways to trigger leptin resistance. Your body is happiest with daily between-meal periods of no food and substantial exertion.

Adiponectin hormone closely mirrors your insulin response. Converse to leptin, if you have more body fat, you should have lower adiponectin. Adiponectin helps insulin work better, so if you are leaner and have higher adiponectin, you can get by with lower insulin. To review, *your goal is to be insulin-sensitive,* which means that a little insulin in your bloodstream gets the glucose put away just fine. If insulin's helper, adiponectin, is not around, more insulin is required, which of course makes more fat. Here comes the positive feedback again. Adiponectin may be one of the reasons why insulin resistance can be caused by going above the threshold of body fat percentage, over 32 percent in women and over 28 percent in men.

Why not test adiponectin or leptin levels? The values are not well established yet, and furthermore, problems related to these hormones simply mirror your level of fitness and insulin resistance.[32] *They are resultant hormones, not causative.* This means that as you correct the parameters within The Blood Code Progress Panel, especially the HOMA-IR, your leptin and adiponectin function has improved.

Glucagon and Cortisol

Glucagon reinforces that meals are meant to pay back what you have used; what you just ate at a meal is for storage. Glucagon opposes the action of insulin. Your body is a two-footed driver, apparently, with the most sophisticated slip clutch in the world. Take a minute to appreciate the elegance of your system . . .

Okay, back to the hormone talk. The law of homeostasis is at work here. If, in response to insulin, you were to put away too much glucose, you could be in trouble. The very gland that makes insulin to move glucose out of the bloodstream contrarily secretes the hormone glucagon to release extra glucose for the bloodstream. Unless a drug effect is involved, like excess injected insulin, your body does not allow you to die from low blood sugar; instead, it quickly and smartly resolves the issue with the release of numerous hormones, like glucagon and cortisol. Under stress, your body releases glucagon, assuming that you will need some extra glucose to support your fight or flight; cortisol is a related stress hormone.

Cortisol is released by a different gland, the adrenal (suprarenal) gland. When you respond to stress, the fight-or-flight experience results from an adrenal release of the neurotransmitters, epinephrine and norepinephrine, formerly known as adrenaline and noradrenaline. The adrenal gland also releases the hormone cortisol, to help sustain the higher adrenaline (fight-or-flight response). Like glucagon, cortisol does the opposite of insulin: It signals for the release of glucose from tissue, not the storage. It also allows muscles to break down (catabolism), assuming that the explosive action of muscles is more important to survive the moment; rebuilding (anabolism) can happen some other day—if there is another day.

Much has been written about how this system is best used for short bouts of stress that benefit from explosive action, with a longer period of recovery to follow.[33] Although many modern stresses are not of the physical body—job change, divorce, financial stresses—they all trigger the same old stress response, just as though you were being physically threatened in the short term. There will often be weight loss during a time of high stress, a result of muscle loss and lack of recovery. The same happens when ill-advised people pursue "weight-loss" treatments that utilize stimulant medication, such as phentermine or other off-label uses of stimulant amphetamine medications. You might even know someone who has lost twenty pounds going through a really stressful divorce; you don't look at them and say, "Hey, you look great!" Something is different about their weight loss; because it is actually muscle loss, there is an emaciated appearance and underlying weakness and fatigue that is evident even to the untrained eye.

Cortisol gets unnecessarily blamed for causing resistant abdominal fat. "Reduce cortisol and belly fat" is an oft-repeated article on the Internet. This section will help you confidently navigate this marketing-rich world.

So here goes; let's look at what cortisol does for you in a typical day:

1) *Cortisol releases upon rising from a night's sleep.* In fact, the most stressful thing you will do in the course of a day, if measured by cortisol release, is wake up. Your morning cortisol allows a release of sugars to fuel your brain and body at a time when, without food, your body is heating up for the day.

2) *Cortisol releases when you exercise.* This is no surprise, since cortisol is a fight-or-flight hormone. When you move your body in a fight-or-flight pattern, cortisol releases to fuel the effort.

3) *Cortisol releases when you eat.* This one is harder to understand, since insulin also releases when you eat. Why would your body release the very hormone that seemingly contradicts the actions of insulin? Like glucagon, this goes back to "why we eat." The food you consume at a meal is best used to repair and re-store what has been drawn upon over prior hours/days. The vast majority of what you eat is not meant to provide energy for future hours; it is to pay back debt. So cortisol provides some glucose from your storage, which allows the foods you just ate to become part of your body structure. Another well-established theory is that cortisol is released at mealtimes because the act of eating and digesting is a pro-inflammatory act in your body, so the anti-inflammatory action of cortisol is desirable.

4) *Cortisol releases under perceived psychosocial stress.* The key word here is *perceived*. It doesn't matter what is actually going on in your life, as much as how you perceive and respond to it. With all the hormonally stressful things that you endure in a day— waking up, eating, and exercising—it's important to have some daily activities that will reduce the effects of stress and allow your body to restore and recover to a calmer baseline. Suffice to say that cortisol is not some evil hormone that is "causing" your body to accrue fat; rather, it's a desirable hormone that fluctuates with your daily demands. Some stress-reduction solutions are found in the prior chapter, "Lifestyle Habits."

Hormones in perspective, not in a pill: Be cautious of any program that claims that taking a pill will improve your hormones. With over sixty-five hormones in the body—and countless other chemical compounds that have local, hormone-like effects, each creating a change in all the others through positive and negative feedback on both central and peripheral tissues—it is mathematically inconceivable that the addition of a chemical hormone to the body can have a single predictable effect. For us humans, our food, fitness, nutrition, mindfulness, and environment have a more-predictable impact on our hormonal balance than the power of any pill.

Whew. This review of hormones can be a little exhausting, but it needs to be discussed, since we are all inundated with continuous advertisements about hormones and weight gain and the miracle pill that will be your savior. If you were looking for the one-pill-easy-fix for your metabolism, you would have stopped reading this book by now.

Thank you for reading, and for taking the self-directed interest in yourself and your metabolic future. It will pay great dividends in your future.

Meal Planner and Guide

I have written this book to help you learn how to guide your own personal lifestyle habits, to allow you to live in accordance with your health potential. Recipes and meals will obviously be part of your journey. I personally own eighty different cookbooks, and I use about three of them, only a few times per year at that.

At a recent conference, I was talking to a twenty-four-year-old PhD nutrition student at Duke University. She said that she didn't own a single cookbook, and couldn't figure out why she would ever need one. She said she eats mostly local and mostly "paleo," which is to say that she eats little fruit, no grains, and little to no sugar. Her meals are simple: some protein, and two to four vegetables, some cooked, some fermented, and only a few raw. "It's pretty simple," she said.

So there you go; it's pretty easy. This recipe chapter will be more about helpful hints to get you started on the path toward easy, intuitive eating. TheBloodCode.com has a forum for recipes and ideas from the community of people that are successfully working toward living within their genetic tolerance. You can further develop your dietary plan based upon your own needs, so visit the site to access the many useful cooking and meal tips that will help balance your unique Blood Code Diet.

Three Effective Breakfasts, Lunches, and Dinners

BREAKFAST

Many people are not very hungry at breakfast time, yet studies repeatedly show that those who eat breakfast have better blood sugar control and concentration and mood throughout the day. So what's the scoop?

A burst of adrenaline and cortisol occurs as you wake from sleeping; in part, this is to prepare you for the most stressful part of your day: getting out of bed. It is also to generate some body heat, since it is normal for your temperature to drop 1 to 2 degrees overnight while sleeping. All of this neurochemical stimulation in your body—called the *dawn phenomenon*—raises your blood sugar and lowers your appetite. With this in mind, you can understand why you need a lower carb intake at breakfast compared to your other meals.

Your first meal needs to be designed to repair and replace the tissue lost during the prior ten- to twelve-hour fast. This means you need to eat a smart meal in the morning. It doesn't need to be a lot if you aren't hungry, but it needs to be something.

Here are three basic breakfasts, all of which can be modified to fit your time frame and cuisine preferences. Even those with no insulin resistance should limit carbs to 30 to 40 grams at the first meal of the day. For reference, a banana and bowl of granola is over 60 grams of carb.

Breakfast #1: Eggs and Veggies

What: Two eggs, any dark leafy greens, fat of your choice, and a piece of toast that matches your carb tolerance.

How: Put your fat of choice into a pan (olive oil, butter, or a high-quality rendered animal fat). Cook the eggs the way you like, ensuring that there's enough fat to sauté the greens in the same pan. Salt to taste. Toast a tolerable amount of bread and butter it well.

Carb count: About 2 grams for the greens; half a piece of toast has 6 to 12 grams of carb; 0 grams for eggs and dietary fats.

Calorie talk: Eggs have 180 calories; 20 for greens; 40 to 50 for toast. Each Tbsp of butter or olive oil has 90 to 100 calories, so add 2 Tbsp of dietary fats to bring your breakfast to a satisfying 400 to 450 calories. Let's say your daily goal is about 2,000 calories; you are getting only 20 percent of your calories with this breakfast, so, as expected, it is your smallest meal of the day.

Bread substitute: Oven-roasted veggies (a hearty mix of carrots, parsnips, cauliflower, onions, and garlic—even potatoes, if you can tolerate more carbs) can be roasted ahead of time with ample olive oil and butter and reheated as needed. They are even good cold. A sprinkle of Parmesan cheese adds a lot of flavor. A good 3-ounce serving will be only 5 to 10 grams of carb, and it offers far more nutrition than bread.

Breakfast #2: Dairy-Based

What: 4 ounces whole-fat, plain yogurt,* ten to twelve almonds, cashews, or pecans

How: No further preparation required.

Carb count: About 7 grams for the yogurt, 1 for the nuts.

Calorie talk: The yogurt has 80 calories, the nuts, 100. This is a snack-like breakfast with only 200 calories, or one-tenth of a 2,000-calorie diet. This is a very small breakfast on its own.

Yogurt substitute: Cottage cheese for yogurt for lower carb and higher protein, this due to the addition of dry milk solids in the cottage cheese. You might also add a hard-boiled egg and greens to this meal for extra calories and no extra carbs.

* *You can easily make your own yogurt, as I do; I also add extra cream into the milk before heating/cooling and pitching the yogurt starter. This makes a higher-fat and lower-carb food for half the cost of yogurt. Learn how to make your own yogurt at TheBloodCode.com.*

Breakfast #3: Meat-Based

I grew up with some Italian cuisine, and I recall that it was always a big deal during Lent to give up meat for one day per week, Friday. Generations ago, my Italian ancestors probably had some meat at nearly every meal, so to avoid meat (and eat only fish, not considered meat) for a full twenty-four hours was considered a worthy sacrifice within the Catholic community. (Sicily has a disproportionate number of people over a hundred years old, and, as with other parts of the world, it appears as though this is partially diet-related.)

How far we have come. Maybe it's time to bring some nutrient-dense meat back to breakfast, especially if you are active and require significant carb restriction.

Quebecois French: Two Wasa (or similar) crackers with spreadable pâté. In our area of Maine, *cretons* (pronounced "creh-tohn") is a spreadable pork pâté that makes a good breakfast or predinner snack.

Any leftovers from dinner: Pork, chicken, beef, fish—sauté a little meat in some olive oil and add whatever greens you have on hand. If fresh veggies are hard to come by, prewashed spinach, kale, or other cooking greens are available in nearly every food market. Eat with toast or the roasted veggies listed in Breakfast #1.

Carb count: None for the meat or pâté; the greens are about 2 grams per cup of cooked greens, so the cracker, bread, or roasted root veggies are the only carbs that need to be counted.

Calorie talk: Meats are dense; this means they have more nutrition and more calories per forkful, which is desirable when you need to get enough sustenance without feeling full.

Substitutions: The options are endless. Many people at my office have successfully reversed their diabetes by eating nontraditional meals at breakfast, like chicken soup or meat and veggie leftovers. This is an effective way to avoid the unfortunately popular grains, fruit, and sugar that dominate even the "healthy choice" boxed cereal breakfasts.

LUNCH

Many workplaces offer little time for lunch, and few people go home for lunch anymore. Meals are often eaten at a desk (which I did for the past twenty years so I wouldn't have to spend the late evening hours making calls and doing charts) or purchased out. Either way, simple and easy choices can provide you with an adequate carbohydrate balance. I am no stranger to having limited time to eat, but there is no room for excuses when aiming for your best health.

Lunch #1: Pack from Home

Leftovers.

I'm tempted to just end it there. This means that your evening meal should always be cooked with extra protein and veggies. When cleaning up from dinner, put a "leftovers" meal together in one of those Pyrex, or similar, glass containers. These are excellent for storage and travel and can be put directly into an oven if needed.

What if I have no leftovers? I'll usually have extra veggies made ahead of time, like roasted root vegetables or coleslaw. I can then grab a can of tuna or wild salmon or sardines. These are quick proteins if you have a taste for them. You can then add some aged cheese and cracker according to your preference for a sustainable meal.

The French Picnic: In a pinch, with no leftovers, I will simply pack a lunch from the veggie and cheese / cured meat drawers in the refrigerator. A little cracker or bread, some nuts, a chunk of naturally cured meat, a chunk of cheese, a pickle /fresh snap peas / radishes / or other raw veggies and some pitted black olives.

Carb count: A bowl of leftovers can look confusing when you're trying to count the carbs, but remember, staple carbs (see page 117) provide insignificant carbs compared to the starchy ones. The 3 to 5 grams of carbs from kale, onions, and pieces of carrots in a chicken stew are negligible compared to the rice in the bowl. At 10 grams of carbs per 4 Tbsp of rice, or 10 grams of carbs per egg-sized potato, you can count up to your personalized carb range with these starchy additions.

Calorie talk: The dietary fats that are typically included in a dinner meal will help this lunch provide you with meaningful calories for your day. As I said earlier in this book, when you eat your larger meal of the day—midday or evening—doesn't matter in terms of your weight and metabolism; it's up to you and your lifestyle.

Lunch #2: Eat Out, Fast

Fast-food places should be avoided. The proteins are usually too processed and then placed between an exorbitant amount of bread. Find an establishment that can accommodate your needs.

Sandwich without bread: Virtually any deli that makes sandwiches can make a platter that has a bed of lettuce, salad dressing, and a mix of other veggies and meats.

Protein: Chicken salad, turkey salad, pulled pork, egg salad, any in-house roasted meat, smoked fish, or a hamburger.

Veggies: Take any veggies, raw or cooked, and top with salad dressing or olive oil. Some nuts and cheese on the salad add a nice crunch and texture, with low-carb nutrients.

Starchy carb: You can then add the amount of carb to your tolerance, such as potato salad or a cracker.

Soup and stew can effectively replace a sandwich and provide a to-go vehicle for meats and vegetables.

Carb count: Sandwich bread is ubiquitous at quick lunches. Each piece delivers 14 to 20 grams per slice. *If your goal is to stay below 20 grams of carbs at lunch, simply remove the extra bread to bring you into your carb range.*

Calorie talk: Two pieces of bread equals 200 calories, so if you remove the bread and forego a sandwich, you may need to replace the calories, or the meal will not satisfy you. The 200 calories is found in an avocado or twenty pecan halves, or a combination of 1 Tbsp mayonnaise and ten cashews or almonds.

Lunch #3: Eat Out, Slow

Once you sit down in a restaurant, you no longer need the hand-grabbing convenience of the bun or wrap or sandwich bread. Restaurant menus usually offer salads as an alternative to a sandwich. If you need to significantly limit bread and carbs, I suggest you ask for twice the dressing for your salad. If you don't get enough fats to sustain you, you will be noticeably hungry only a few hours later. Get a side of olives instead of bread if you want something to munch ahead of time.

Ethnic eating offers an incredible resource that helps you move away from the sandwich and chips habit in the United States.

Asian, rice-based meals: Vietnamese pho is a mix of noodles with meat, veggies, and a wildly nutritious and flavorful broth. The lunch menu in a Thai restaurant is virtually all meat or fish and vegetables. You add the quantity of rice you can tolerate. Chinese meals are the same if you avoid the sweet sauces and fried foods; you will be able to regulate your carbohydrate based on your rice intake (4 Tbsp rice contains about 10 grams of carb).

Mexican: I never get burritos out because the wrap itself is about 60 grams of carb, and then it's stuffed with rice and beans; this could throw me back into prediabetes within weeks. But if I eat *in* the burrito shop, I can get the modified burrito bowl: a bed of spinach, a small scoop of hot beans, pork/beef/chicken/fish, shredded lettuce, tomatoes, onions, and avocado. This fabulous meal eliminates the convenient (but carbo-loaded) wrap and turns it into a better fork-and-knife meal.

DINNER

For those of you who eat a quicker, more incidental lunch, the evening meal becomes even more important, since it might comprise nearly half of your calories for the day. People who have successfully corrected their Blood Code often share the same dinner/meal secret. Are you ready for this? *You can have more than one vegetable with dinner.*

It's simple: Your old, meat, vegetable, and potato/bread/pasta meal can be modified to meat, vegetable, vegetable, vegetable.

Dinner #1: "I didn't prepare and don't have time."

For this meal, find a protein that you can cook quickly (preprepared vegetables are helpful).

Meats: Beef tips or hamburger (get the highest fat content possible) are ready in a pan in only 10 minutes. Chicken typically takes longer, but this might be a time to go for a boneless skin-on chicken thigh for the pan.

Thin filets of fish: Cover with butter, herbs, and lemon slices and bake or broil until it flakes (usually in only 5 minutes). *Salad:* This can be as simple as the lettuce of your choice, or with added vegetables. Use the dressing listed at the end of this chapter.

Steamed vegetables: Broccoli and/or carrots cut lengthwise, or asparagus, or any other vegetable that brightens and softens when steamed. Done within 5 minutes; add olive oil or butter.

Sautéed vegetables: If you have cooked steak tips or hamburger, you will have the drippings in the pan. Add butter or olive oil to the drippings and quick-sauté any "tougher" vegetable, like string beans, mushrooms, fennel, onions, garlic, snow peas, or the dark leafy greens (collards/chard/kale). You won't be baking a squash for this meal, because you're in a hurry, remember?

Dinner #2: "I have time earlier in the day to prepare."

Meat/fish/chicken: Buy any bone-in cut you can find. Recover the fats and nutrient-rich juices that cook out.

Bone-in pork roast / bone-in beef roast / bone-in lamb roast: Sear the outside with a heat-tolerant fat, like lard or ghee. Olive oil will also work here. This is messy without a screen cover; get it to snap-crackle-pop. Once all sides are browned—this will take a total of 10 minutes—place in a covered oven-roasting pot. (I do my browning and slow-cooking in the same Creuset pan—less to clean.) Set the oven at about 250 degrees Fahrenheit and roast for four to six hours. This cooking method is called a "braise," and Crock-Pots are designed for this purpose. The minerals and nutrients inside the bone cook into the meat and juices.

Whole chicken can be done in a similar fashion, without the browning, and the bird will only need about four hours. Make sure it is covered well, in a Creuset, clay pot, or in a pan with foil. Uncover at the end if you want it browned a little.

Fish: Look for a whole fish; this takes some time to take apart once cooked, but remember, this is a meal for when you have time.

Roasted root vegetables: About 30 to 60 minutes before the meal, put root vegetables (onions, carrots, potatoes, parsnips, or pieces of turnip and winter squash) in the pot with the roast; they will cook in the nutritious juices. Remember that the carrots and turnips have less than a third the carb content as potatoes for the same volume, so choose the lower-carb root veggies listed in Step Four, Dietary Carbohydrates (see page 118).

Just before the meal, put together a salad. Lay out a plate of raw veggies as a side dish—like radishes, snap peas, or cucumber—to balance out the warming, hearty flavors of the slow-cooked braise.

Again, we have the same theme: meat, veggie, veggie, veggie. And remember, make too much; the main course will provide leftovers for an excellent lunch in upcoming days.

Dinner #3: "I'm eating out."

The rules of eating out for dinner are the same as they are for lunch. Eliminate the pre-meal bread; this will prevent your insulin from going up even before the meal arrives. Dinner does offer an extra challenge over lunch: alcohol. This was discussed in the earlier "Lifestyle Habits" chapter, and should be respected for both the carb content of the alcoholic beverage, and the fat storage effect that the alcohol triggers.

Most every restaurant, even though the option may not be listed on the menu, will offer an extra serving of vegetables instead of pasta/potato/rice. Even the barbecue restaurants in New England offer side dishes of stewed collards and pickled okra. I can always find a balanced meal trading in the corn bread for some coleslaw and greens. Enjoy.

Your personal cuisine should play a significant role in how you apply the principles of The Blood Code Diet; therefore, your dietary success will look very different from that of a person from a different culture or cuisine. The conversation needs to be ongoing. TheBloodCode.com has a nutritional forum, which includes recipes, ideas, and solutions from our staff and the community of people following the steps of The Blood Code. Visit the website, sign up for the newsletter, and become part of the conversation. Among other things, you'll learn how to make your own high-fat yogurt, how to tenderize kale by freezing, and what to look for in sauerkraut.

Sample Recipe from TheBloodCode.com
Real Salad Dressing

Most store-bought dressing includes cheap vegetable oils. The quality you will enjoy from a good bottle of olive oil is beyond comparison. Let's keep it really simple. I make one salad dressing 95 percent of the time, so let's do that one first.

In a separate jar or in the bottom of your salad bowl, before the lettuce goes in, mix together extra virgin, cold-pressed, first-pressed olive oil; lemon juice (fresh); Celtic salt; and Dijon mustard. That's it. You should use at least 2 to 3 ounces of olive oil to accommodate the juice of one lemon, but if you, like me, need extra non-carb calories, go heavy on the olive oil.

The other 5 percent of the time, I make Caesar salad dressing. This is the same as above, with one change: Add an egg yolk to the lemon juice first; whip together, then slowly add the olive oil while whipping. When it thickens slightly, add the other ingredients. This is served with romaine lettuce, anchovies, and pecorino Romano or aged Parmesan cheese.

Staying in Your Sweet Spot

To improve is to change; to be perfect is to change often.
—Winston Churchill

The changes you make in your diet, fitness, and nutrition habits will need to adjust over time. To stay fit, research shows that you actually need to work a little harder and smarter as you age in order to maintain the same fitness level. So, too, if you had insulin resistance early in your life, you will need to be more diligent with your diet decades later.[1] A good perspective will help you. If you view each change as a burden caused by the injustice of disease, you are doomed. Remember that the reason you make diet and fitness changes is not because of some disease that you caught; it is to live in accordance with your brilliant expression of survival and being.

It can be said again that insulin resistance is not something you *have*; it is something that *is happening*. You are prepared for survival by having traits that help you to perform a lot of physical activity while also being resistant to famine. It is up to you to live up to these excellent traits and not ignore them. You may be told that you *have* a cholesterol problem, or that you *have* high blood pressure. Don't get stuck with the stigma of disease ownership. It is true that as you become insulin-resistant, your blood pressure will go up. But it is just as true that as you correct your insulin resistance, your blood pressure will go down. Many of your symptoms are only temporal events that occur given your current diet, fitness, and nutritional status. Change the conditions in the right direction for you, and you will reap the reward of wellness.

Be in touch with your prescribing health-care provider if you are on medication: If you are managed on any medication for blood pressure or blood sugar, you will need to check in with your health-care provider when you start to follow the steps of The Blood Code. Medications to address lipid problems, blood pressure, and blood sugar will typically need to be reduced or removed as you more appropriately and more effectively "treat" yourself with your self-guided diet and fitness habits.

I am all for skepticism, so retest your Blood Code panel when you want an objective assessment of your progress. Monitor blood pressure with a qualified provider, and check your body fat changes with your skin-fold calipers at home. As stated at the beginning of this book, you do not need to "believe" in the steps of The Blood Code, but you *do* need to believe in yourself.

To begin, plot your health coordinates with your Blood Code Discovery Panel. Take a ninety-day challenge, or longer if you can maintain your self-prescribed changes, and retest with the Progress Panel. From there, an annual check of the blood test will usually be adequate. Once you have two to three coordinates on your health map, you will better know the path you are on and the habits you need to maintain or improve upon.

I realize that there are still anxious eaters around you who might "believe" that a diet rich in saturated fats is harmful, no matter what the evidence suggests. As a skeptic, I am always prepared to be wrong or to see another idea or reason for something, so I too rely on the progress of science and prevailing evidence provided by rational interpretation of research. Visit TheBloodCode.com and sign up for our newsletter and private forum for clinical questions that will provide you with the personalized support and reinforcement you will need along the way. Free resources at the website and in the newsletters will also provide timely and useful insights for you and those around you.

Pat yourself on the back; you have accepted something about your genetics and lifestyle—your very being—that perfectly shape you for this moment. You have addressed your food, fitness, and nutritional habits with a firm confidence and self-awareness. You own your accomplishments. This is not some fad diet or exercise program that you tried for a while, and then abandoned. You are moving toward a future of healthier being.

I am sure you realize that perfection is only momentary; you need to constantly adjust and renew your efforts. Your friends and family can help you do this, and I hope this book and website can help you, too. Retest your Blood Code Panel and skin-fold caliper measurements to ensure that you are on the right path.

Thanks for allowing TheBloodCode team to be part of your journey.

—Dr. Richard Maurer

Glossary

THE BLOOD CODE GLOSSARY

Adiponectin: This hormone—along with its sister hormone, leptin—is released from fat cells in your body, and plays a part in the regulation of your blood sugar and metabolism. Adiponectin helps insulin to work better; it makes you more insulin-sensitive. Inversely, the lower your body fat percentage, the higher your adiponectin levels, and the more insulin-sensitive you are. It follows that as your body fat content goes up, your adiponectin level drops, leaving you more insulin-resistant.

Anabolism / anabolic: The metabolic process that builds complex tissue like fat or muscle. Energy is stored within these tissues and is released only when the complex structures are broken down into simpler form. (See below for more on *catabolism*.)

Basal body temperature (BBT) / Basal metabolic rate (BMR): Your baseline (or first-thing-in-the-morning) body temperature. The measurable heat represents, in part, the rate of biological processes at work—your basal metabolic rate, or BMR.

Body fat percentage: The relative portion of your total weight that is composed from fatty tissue. Skin-fold calipers offer the practiced individual the ability to calculate body fat percentage with simple charts. By extension, the remaining percentage of your body weight is made up of bone, muscle, connective tissue, etc.

Carbohydrate code: The term used in this book to help you find your unique carbohydrate tolerance with current blood test results and skin-fold caliper measurements.

Catabolism / catabolic: The opposite (but equal metabolic process) of *anabolism,* where complex tissues are broken down to simpler form. Stored energy is released when complex tissues such as body fat are broken down. Processes like body fat gain and fatty liver result when your catabolic activity is inadequate to balance your anabolic gains.

Complex carbohydrate: The class of foods that deliver glucose from long-chain starches, as compared to short, one- and two-chain sugars that are called *simple carbohydrates.* Complex carbohydrates include both kale and white flour, exemplifying the different carb and fiber content possible in this category.

Cortisol: This hormone comes from a portion of your adrenal gland in response to the daily stresses of life. The actions of this hormone are so many that it defies the label of "friend" or "foe" (good or bad). Instead, cortisol defines the complex effect that stress, of all kinds, has on your mind and body.

Dawn phenomenon: Your blood sugar will rise, without food or drink, in the first few hours of your day. Regardless of the stressful things you might encounter later on, getting out of bed is the most biochemically stressful moment in your day. Remember: Your body is prepared for a more physically demanding world with few easily available calories.

Epigenetics: The study of the ability to change genetic expression without changing the DNA itself. The study of epigenetics describes why many disease conditions—like insulin resistance, in particular—are not well explained by simple genetics. Lifestyle, environment, and diet are effectively able to switch gene expression on or off.

Fasting glucose / fasting blood sugar: The measurement of your blood glucose without the influence of food or calories from the prior ten to twelve hours, usually overnight.

Fatty liver disease: Over the years, complicated medical terms have described this condition, including *nonalcoholic steatohepatitis* (NASH) and *benign hepatic steatosis. Fatty liver* is more apt, referring to the excessive fat that accumulates in the liver, frequently accompanied by the triad of high blood pressure, elevated liver enzymes, and high triglycerides.

Glipizide (brand name Glucotrol): This is the most common drug that a conventional doctor will add, after Metformin, to lower blood sugars. The action of this Sulfonylurea class of drugs is to trigger your pancreas to release *more* insulin. While this will lower your blood sugar, the very problem of insulin resistance is complicated by this drug mechanism.

Glucagon: A hormone, like insulin, which is secreted from the pancreas yet has an opposite reaction. Glucagon causes increased blood glucose through the release of stored sugars in your liver.

Glycemic index: An overly simplistic attempt to categorize foods by the speed and extent that blood glucose elevates following a specific carbohydrate food. The sugar fructose has a delayed but disastrous effect on overall blood sugar control, yet because the glucose onset is delayed, it remains low on the glycemic index.

Goitrogens: By pure definition, any substance that induces an enlargement of the thyroid gland, or goiter. Some foods have goitrogenic properties that especially affect people with iodine deficiency. The goitrogenic activity of foods like broccoli and cabbage is removed with cooking.

Hashimoto's thyroiditis: The most common process by which hypothyroidism occurs. Thyroid peroxidase (TPO) antibodies, if activated, can decrease overall thyroid function by reducing a functional portion of the thyroid gland.

Hereditary hemochromatosis: A genetic condition that predisposes an individual to store more iron than usual, marked by elevated ferritin levels. Mild forms of the trait may not require special treatment, whereas severe forms can cause aggressive liver and inflammatory disease if left untreated.

Hyperglycemia / high blood sugar / high blood glucose: When blood glucose is above established normal reference ranges: Fasting blood glucose greater than 100 mg/dL and hemoglobin A1C levels greater than 5.7 percent both designate high blood sugar. *Insulin resistance* is the mechanism by which fasting blood sugars begin to rise over time.

Hyperthyroidism: The state where the thyroid gland produces an excess of thyroid hormones, or where prescription thyroid hormone medication is excessive. A TSH below normal typically indicates a hyperthyroid process.

Hypoglycemia / low blood sugar / low blood glucose: Under normal circumstances, low blood sugar is not a medical concern because the body can quickly release hormones, like glucagon, to help elevate the blood sugar to normal. Those who take insulin or medications that raise insulin levels are at risk of problematic episodes of low blood sugar.

Hypothyroidism: The state where there is inadequate thyroid hormone in the body, or where there is inadequate thyroid hormone activation. An elevated TSH is a likely finding, but does not define the condition.

Insulin resistance (IR): This is the umbrella term that describes your body's ability to contain blood glucose with a reasonably normal insulin level. The HOMA-IR calculation quantifies the extent of any insulin resistance.

Insulin sensitivity: This is your goal: A small amount of total insulin effectively keeps your blood sugars under tight control. Disease prevention and longevity are associated with insulin sensitivity, measured by a low HOMA-IR of 1 or less.

Leptin: Like adiponectin, leptin is released from your fat cells, and in a perfect world, it turns off your hunger. The more fat cells you have, the more leptin will be released; as a result, your body will experience less hunger at that moment.

Metabolic syndrome / Reaven's syndrome / MetSyn / MetS: A constellation of different symptoms that all result from underlying insulin resistance. It is defined by having several of the following indicators: elevated abdominal body fat, borderline / high blood pressure, low HDL, elevated triglyceride, elevated blood glucose. It is well established as a risk factor for the development of many chronic degenerative diseases. Prolific researcher Gerald Reaven, of Stanford University in California, was instrumental in establishing the basis of what we now call *metabolic syndrome*.

Metabolism: This term is best defined as the rate of biological processes in an organism. In human health, the word *metabolism* describes the processes of anabolism and catabolism, or the storing and releasing of energy.

Metformin (brand name Glucophage): This is the number-one drug used to lower blood sugar or to address insulin resistance, with a pill. It remains the go-to drug because it does not raise insulin, a mechanism that appears to come with dire consequences when relied upon to normalize blood glucose.

"Paleo" (Paleolithic) diets: Paleo diets are a popular way to frame food choices that mimic what might have been available to humans more than 10,000 years ago, when the Paleolithic era ended; basically, no fruit, legumes, grains, or dairy were available. It is evident that many of us have evolved to tolerate these "new" foods. For most Paleo eaters, the diet becomes low-carb. Those with moderate to severe insulin resistance will find many useful food options in Paleo diet resources.

Polycystic ovary syndrome (PCOS): A condition that is typically found in young women, and where insulin resistance is strongly associated, if not causative. This condition heralds the need to follow the steps outlined in The Blood Code, beginning with the appropriate blood tests (The Discovery Panel).

Prediabetes / prediabetic: No one reaches type 2 diabetes without being prediabetic for years, if not decades. The focus of this book is to offer you the tools you need to identify this pattern as early as possible, when some easy steps can fully reverse the process before it ever takes root in your metabolism.

Satiety: The satisfaction you feel following a meal. The more a meal promotes satiety (e.g., a meal that is rich in saturated fats), the less you will experience cravings and the *need* to snack afterward.

Simple carbohydrates: Aka, simple sugars, monosaccharides, disaccharides, and what are referred to on food labels as simply "sugars." This carbohydrate class of foods includes table sugar (sucrose), milk sugar (lactose), fruit sugar (fructose), malt sugar (maltose), corn sugar (dextrose), and several others. These sugars create unique challenges to your glucose control, and, in excess, are uniquely implicated in the onset of insulin resistance.

Skin-fold calipers: A device that offers a simple way to measure, in millimeters, a pinched area of skin and the attached body fat. Four body locations uniquely identify the metabolic response to your diet and exercise.

Type 2 diabetes: The later stage of insulin resistance, where blood glucose levels have reached a tipping point according to our medical diagnostic criteria: The fasting glucose is over 125 mg / dL; the hemoglobin A1C is greater than 6.4 percent; or you experience an after-meal glucose above 200 mg / dL.

Vitamin D: Vitamin D breaks from the typical definition of a vitamin; it's a steroid compound that is both a nutrient and can also be synthesized through your skin, with UVB exposure. Vitamin D deficiency can exacerbate insulin resistance, and, as with other nutrient deficiencies, should be prevented with a rational, moderate supplement plan.

Your Blood Code Charts, Logs, and Worksheets

Test Date:					
Triglyceride, mg/dL					
HDL, mg/dL					
* TG:HDL ratio					
Glucose, mg/dL					
Insulin, uIU/mL					
* HOMA-IR (GxI÷405)					
HgbA1C, %					
ALT enzyme					
Vitamin D					
Ferritin					
TSH					
Free T4					
Free T3					
Other Tests:					

*For these calculations, use U.S. standard units

Your goal for TG:HDL and HOMA-IR is a value of about 1.
TG:HDL ratio is simply a division of TG/HDL.
HOMA-IR is Glucose (in mg/dL) X Insulin (in uIU/mL) ÷ 405.
If you are starting in non-U.S. (S.I. units), use the Table of Units Conversion or visit TheBloodCode.com for these and other resources.

The Blood Code: Table of Units Conversion

Test Name	U.S. standard unit	Conversion Factor For U.S. to S.I. → multiply For S.I. to U.S. ← divide	Standard International (S.I.)
WBC	%	0.01	unit of 1
Hemoglobin (Hgb)	g/dL	10	g/L
Hematocrit (Hct)	%	0.01	unit of 1
BUN	mg/dL	0.357	mmol/L
Creatinine	mg/dL	88.4	umol/dL
Glucose	mg/dL	0.0556	mmol/L
Insulin	uIU/mL	6.0	pmol/L
HgbA1c	%	[%-2.15] * 10.9	mmol/mol
Triglyceride (TG)	mg/dL	0.011	mmol/L
HDL cholesterol	mg/dL	0.026	mmol/L
Total cholesterol	mg/dL	0.026	mmol/L
Ferritin	ng/mL	1	ug/L
Vitamin D	ng/mL	2.5	nmol/L
TSH	uIU/mL	1	mIU/L
Free T4	ng/dL	12.9	pmol/L
Free T3	pg/dL	0.015	pmol/L

Liver enzymes AST and ALT along with other components of the complete blood count (CBC) such as MCV, MCH and platelets are identical between systems.

HGB A1C Conversion Chart

U.S. Standard: %	S.I.: mmol/mol
4.5	26
5.0	31
5.5	36
5.7	39
5.9	41
6.1	43
6.3	45
6.5	47
7.0	53
7.5	58
8.0	64

Skin-fold caliper measurements with their total:

DATE →						
TRICEPS						
BICEPS						
BACK						
HIP						
Total mm						
Body fat %						

*Your goal is Triceps = Back = Hip (within 3 to 5 mm)

The Blood Code Body Fat Evaluation Table

For Women			For Men		
TOTAL MM		BODY FAT %	TOTAL MM		BODY FAT %
14–15	Too Low	12	12–13	Too Low	7
16–17		14	14–15		8
18–19		15	16–17		9
20–21	Below Normal	17	20–21	Below Normal	11
22–23		18	22–23		12
24–25		19	24–25		13
26–27	Normal	20	26–27	Normal	14
28–29		21	27–28		15
30–34		22	29–31		16
35–39		23	32–35		17
40–44		25	36–38		18
45–49		26	39–42		19
50–54		28	43–45		20
55–59		29	46–49		21
60–64		30	50–54		22
65–69	Too High	31	55–59	Too High	23
70–74		32	60–65		24
75–79		33	66–73		25
80–84	Obese	34	74–79	Obese	26
85–89		35	80–85		27
90–94		36	86–91		28
95–99		37	92-98		29
100–109		38	99–105		30
110–119		39	106–115		31
120–129		40	116–125		32
130–139		41	126–135		33
140–150		42	136–145		34
151–160		43	146–156		35

The Blood Code Discussion for Athletes

A future collaboration will cover the many ways to improve your athletic performance through your Blood Code. It is likely that many athletes are not meeting their body's metabolic needs with their meals, snacks, and training techniques. Workout goals regarding insulin are the same as nonathletes: Insulin should be kept low during workouts, and should be in the sweet spot after meals, no higher. Insulin is an anabolic hormone, so it can be a blessing for an athlete's exercise recovery and a curse if too high during the activity.

I have seen well-conditioned endurance athletes with very high triglycerides and high blood pressure. They often carbo-load with processed goos, gels, bars, or smoothies. As you have heard throughout this book, if you find out that you are in the 40 to 50 percent of people that tend toward high insulin or insulin resistance, you do not need the oft-recommended carbo-loads, even during vigorous training. Insulin levels should *not* be high during exercise. Athletes that naturally have higher insulin should restrict carbs before a workout, and should not consider glucose packets and sugar replacement in their longer workouts.

Conversely, I have seen young athletes go on a carb-restricted diet or an overly restrictive "paleo" diet, only to find that they end up tired and not feeling well. If your Blood Code Test Panel reveals insulin of <2, it is *too* low. This means with each workout, you go catabolic—you break down muscle rather than build up strength.

Athletes need adequate insulin release with meals in order to replenish glycogen and build muscle after vigorous exertion; protein stimulates a substantial insulin release, albeit, to a lesser degree than carbohydrates. Those with low insulin will likely need a protein recovery meal within an hour of a vigorous workout, and will also benefit from a starchy carbohydrate at the meal.

Much more can be said about applying The Blood Code for athletes in training, and this will certainly be a future project. For now, I'd recommend that any athlete take the steps to discover their baseline insulin and insulin resistance. This will instruct their dietary habits more effectively than a one-size-fits-all program.

To help you gain more understanding about how your Blood Code can be used to enhance your athletic performance, look for future articles and posts on TheBloodCode.com, and sign up for our newsletters.

TheBloodCode.com Website

The Blood Code™ is a book, clinic, web resource, and community of people, who, like you, are ready to take responsibility for their own wellness, health recovery, and illness prevention. Once empowered by the personal significance of your metabolic blood test results and skin-fold caliper measurements, you can accurately prescribe your own diet, nutrition, and fitness habits and measure the influence on your present health and future. The Team at TheBloodCode.com works to provide a rational and well-researched voice toward dietary, nutritional, and fitness recommendations through our on-location services, retreats, website updates, and forum commentary.

At The Blood Code—Maine, Dr. Maurer and his team can help you interpret the meaning and unique significance that your metabolic blood test results and skin-fold caliper measurements have on your health and longevity. Dr. Maurer leads Metabolic Recovery Retreats that combine metabolic consultations, nutrition and fitness classes, along with hands-on cooking instruction. Information about upcoming retreats can be found at TheBloodCode.com.

Dietary Resources

Through the website, we maintain links to helpful resources, recipes, and food blogs. These resources change often, so a printed list is less useful than a quick visit to the website. Sign up for our free newsletter, or join the forum for a more dynamic question-and-answer format.

Fitness Resources

Our Blood Code Partners at FitnessVideo101 help create fitness modules that support those who are incorporating The Blood Code Fitness Principles. Visit TheBloodCode.com to view some of the current instructional content, more will develop and become available.

Bands and dumbbells can be an effective, if not essential, addition to your home fitness routines. Our website will offer you current information on available and recommended resources for attaining the right products and finding the right instruction.

Dietary and Fitness Referrals

TheBloodCode.com will soon have a listing resource for professionals, nutritional consultants, and trainers familiar with the science, principles, and clinical application of The Blood Code. We hope this list of providers will be an ever-growing resource to find local, hands-on assistance toward your metabolic recovery and health.

Nutrition Resources

Visit TheBloodCode.com for up-to-date nutritional information and access to rational effective nutritional supplements. We at The Blood Code will continue to work on your behalf to cut through the hype and provide genuinely valuable nutritional advice that helps you throughout your healthful journey.

Acknowledgments

Thank you to the many patients and families who have seen me over the past twenty years. The intimacy of a family practice is both inspiring and humbling. I am grateful to those who have shared their health and medical stories; their testimonials on the website and in this book go a long way toward inspiring others to identify and make their own meaningful and self-empowered changes. To the thousands who have made their lives better by following The Blood Code: Advice is worthless without action, so to all, thanks for making my vocation worthwhile.

Thanks to my fellow authors around Portland, Maine, especially Genevieve Morgan, whose assistance was invaluable. Thanks to Patty Hagge and Sarah Corbett, for their writers' eyes and minds. And to all the food and health writers I have come to know through their written stories—they have enriched my quest for health answers over the decades: Andrew Weil, Nina Planck, Michael Pollan, Gretchen Reynolds, Sally Fallon, Gary Taubes, Dr. Richard Bernstein, and Dr. Michael Murray.

Cheers to friend and fellow traveler, Steve Melchiskey, who helped name this manifesto.

I appreciate the vast net of medical colleagues and friends in Maine who provide practice support and helpful dialogue. Thanks to a master trainer, Jeff Eckhouse.

A special thanks to my mother, for her honest and inspiring efforts that have reversed her type 2 diabetes; to my late father, who modeled exercise as a way of life; and to my wife—mother, artist, acupuncturist, coach, friend, and colleague—I am rewarded by all.

And lastly, thanks to you, for finding this book and taking a step toward your deserved health and vitality. Use it well.

Yours,
Dr. Richard Maurer

About the Author

Dr. Richard Maurer, a doctor, author, and parent, has practiced integrative medicine in Maine since 1994. He helps people interpret their unique blood test results to resolve disease and move toward real health and vitality. His own personal and familial trend toward type 2 diabetes has only strengthened his preventive and natural medical pursuits in an effort to help others identify their most effective dietary, nutritional, and fitness habits.

Dr. Maurer has developed TheBloodCode.com to provide a community of empowered men and women who will become experts in their own diet and fitness needs to ensure their longest and healthiest life possible. He travels regularly for lectures and Metabolic Recovery Retreats. Events and more information is found at TheBloodCode.com.

Dr. Maurer earned his doctorate of naturopathic medicine from the National College of Naturopathic Medicine in 1994. His bachelor's degree was in both music performance and chemistry at Temple University in Philadelphia.

Endnotes and Citations

Step One: Get Your Blood Tests

[1] Maratou, E., et al. Studies of insulin resistance in patients with clinical and subclinical hypothyroidism. Eur J Endocrinol. 2009 May; 160(5):785–90.

[2] Ayturk, S. Metabolic syndrome and its components are associated with increased thyroid volume and nodule prevalence in a mild-to-moderate iodine-deficient area. Eur J Endocrinol. 2009 Oct; 161(4):599–605.

[3] Coban, E., et al. Effect of iron deficiency anemia on the levels of hemoglobin A1c in nondiabetic patients. Acta Haematol. 2004; 112(3):126–8.

[4] Sinha, N., Mishra, T. K., Singh, T., Gupta, N. Effect of iron deficiency anemia on hemoglobin A1c levels. Ann Lab Med. 2012; 32:17–22.

[5] Battezzati, A., et al. Effect of hypoglycemia on amino acid and protein metabolism in healthy humans. Diabetes. 2000 Sept., vol. 49; 1543–51.

[6] Emerging Risk Factors Collaboration. Diabetes mellitis, fasting glucose and risk of cause specific death. N Engl J Med. 2011 Mar 3; 364:829–41.

[7] Matsushita, K., et al. The association of hemoglobin A1c with incident heart failure among people without diabetes: The Atherosclerosis Risk in Communities Study. Diabetes. 2010; 59:2020–26.

[8] Staten, M., et al. Insulin Assay Standardization: Leading to Measures of Insulin Sensitivity and Secretion for Practical Clinical Care. Diabetes Care June 2010 vol. 33 no. 6 e84.

[9] da Silva, R. C., et al. Insulin resistance, beta-cell function, and glucose tolerance in Brazilian adolescents with obesity or risk factors for type 2 diabetes mellitus. J Diabetes Compl. 2007 Mar/Apr; 21(2):84–92.

[10] Vogeser, M. Fasting serum insulin and the homeostasis model of insulin resistance (HOMA-IR) in the monitoring of lifestyle interventions in obese persons. Clinical Biochemistry (2007), vol. 40, issue 13/14:964–8.

[11] Kabadi, S., et al. Joint effects of obesity and vitamin D insufficiency on insulin resistance and type 2 diabetes: Results from the NHANES 2001–2006. Diabetes Care. October 2012, vol. 35, no. 10, 2048–54.

[12] Sung, C. C., et al. Role of vitamin D in insulin resistance. J Biomed Biotechnol. 2012; doi: 10.1155/2012/634195.

[13] Vaucher, P., et al. Effect of iron supplementation on fatigue in non-anemic menstruating women with low ferritin. CMAJ, 2012 Aug 7; 184(11):1247–54.

[14] Wrede, C. E., et al. Association between serum ferritin and the insulin resistance syndrome in a representative population. Eur J Endocrinol. 2006 Feb; 154(2):333–40.

[15] Pepys, M. B., Hirschfield, G. M. June 2003. C-reactive protein: A critical update. J Clin Invest, 111 (12):1805–12.

[16] Melander, O., et al. Novel and conventional biomarkers for prediction of incident cardiovascular events in the community. JAMA 2009; 302:49–57.

[17] Maratou, E., et al. Studies of insulin resistance in patients with clinical and subclinical hypothyroidism. Eur J Endocrinol. 2009 May;160(5):785-90.

[18] Ciloglu, F., et al. Exercise intensity and its effects on thyroid hormones. Neuroendocrinology Letters 2005; 26(6):830–4.

[19] Rozing, M. P., et al. Low serum free triiodothyronine levels mark familial longevity: The Leiden Longevity Study. J Gerontol A Biol Sci Med Sci, 2010. 65(4):365–8.

[20] Rozing, M. P., et al. Familial longevity is associated with decreased thyroid function. J Clin Endocrinol Metab, 2010; 95 (11):4979–84.

[21] Maratou, E., et al. Studies of insulin resistance in patients with clinical and subclinical hypothyroidism. Eur J Endocrinol. 2009 May; 160(5):785–90.

Step Two: Measure Yourself with Skin-Fold Calipers

[1] Ostojic, S. M. Estimation of body fat in athletes: Skinfolds vs. bioelectrical impedance. J Sports Med Phys Fitness. 2006 Sep; 46(3):442–6.

Step Three: Putting It All Together—IR, High Insulin, and Hypothyroid

[1] Narayan, K. M. V., et al. Diabetes Care. 2007 June; 30(6) 1562–66.

[2] Xu, Y., et al. Prevalence and control of diabetes in Chinese adults. JAMA. 2013; 310(9):948–59.

[3] Flegal, K. M., et al. Prevalence of obesity and trends in the distribution of body mass index among US adults, 1999–2010. JAMA. 2012; 307(5):491–7.

[4] Yun, K. H., et al. Relationship of thyroid stimulating hormone with coronary atherosclerosis in angina patients. Int J Cardiol 2007; 122(1):56–60.

[5] Maratou, E., et al. Studies of insulin resistance in patients with clinical and subclinical hypothyroidism. Eur J Endocrinol. 2009 May; 160(5):785–90.

[6] Fernández-Real, J. M., et al. Thyroid function is intrinsically linked to insulin sensitivity and endothelium-dependent vasodilation in healthy euthyroid subjects. J Clin Endocrinol Metab 2006; 91(9):3337–43.

[7] Gussekloo, J., et al. Thyroid status, disability and cognitive function, and survival in old age. JAMA 2004; 292(21):2591–99.

[8] Gesing, A., et al. The thyroid gland and the process of aging; what is new? Thyroid Research 2012, 5:16.

[9] Hesse, V., et al. Thyroid hormone metabolism under extreme body exercises. Exp Clin Endocrinol. 1989 Sep; 94(1–2):82–8.

[10] Ciloglu, F., et al. Exercise intensity and its effects on thyroid hormones. Neuroendocrinology Letters 2005 Dec;26(6):830–4.

[11] Fontana, L., et al. Effect of long-term calorie restriction with adequate protein and micronutrients on thyroid hormones. J Clin Endocrinol Metab. 2006 Aug; 91(8):3232–5.

[12] Masterjohn, Chris. http://www.cholesterol-and-health.com/Goitrogen-Special-Report.html

[13] Hackney, A. C., et al. Thyroid hormonal responses to intensive interval versus steady-state endurance exercise sessions. Hormones (Athens). 2012 Jan/Mar; 11(1):54–60.

[14] Kelly, G. Body temperature variability: Masking influences of body temperature variability and a review of body temperature variability in disease. Alt Med Rev. 2007; 12(1):49–62.

Step Four: Adjust Your Blood Code Diet

[1] Holt, S., et al. An insulin index of foods: The insulin demand generated by 1000-kJ portions of common foods. Am J Clin Nutr 1997; 66:1264–76.

[2] Tappy, L., et al. Metabolic effects of fructose and the worldwide increase in obesity. Physiol Rev. 2010 Jan; 90:23–46.

[3] Bocarsly, M. E., et al. High-fructose corn syrup causes characteristics of obesity in rats: Increased body weight, body fat and triglyceride levels. Pharmacol Biochem Behav, 2010 Nov; 97(1):101–6.

[4] Doerge, D. R., Sheehan, D. M. Goitrogenic and estrogenic activity of soy isoflavones. Environ Health Perspect. 2002 Jun; 110 Suppl 3:349–53.

[5] Guyton and Hall. Textbook of Medical Physiology, 12th Edition. Saunders, 2011.

[6] Brown, R., et al. Artificial sweeteners: A systematic review of metabolic effects in youth. Int J Pediatr Obes. 2010 Aug; 5(4):305–12.

[7] Lawrence, G. Dietary fats and health: Dietary recommendations in the context of scientific evidence. Adv Nutr, vol. 4, 2013 May; 294–302.

[8] Tipton, K., Wolfe, R. Protein and amino acids for athletes. Journal of Sports Sciences, 2004; 22, 65–79.

[9] Bernstein, R. Diabetes Solution. Little Brown & Co., 2007.

[10] Layman, D., et al. Increased dietary protein modifies glucose and insulin homeostasis in adult women during weight loss. J. Nutr. 2003 Feb; 133:405–10.

[11] Micha, R. RD, PhD; Wallace, S. K., BA; Mozaffarian, D., MD, DrPH. Red and processed meat consumption and risk of incident coronary heart disease, stroke, and diabetes mellitus. Circulation 2010; 121:2271–83.

[12] Rohrmann, S., et al. Meat consumption and mortality: Results from the European Prospective Investigation into Cancer and Nutrition. BMC Medicine 2013; 11:63.

[13] Paddon-Jones, D., et al. Protein, weight management, and satiety. Am J Clin Nutr. 2008 May; 87(5):1558S–1561S.

[14] Halton, T., et al. The effects of high protein diets on thermogenesis, satiety and weight loss: A critical review. J Am Coll Nutr. 2004 Oct; 23(5):373–85.

[15] Yannakoulia, M., et al. Association of eating frequency with body fatness in pre- and postmenopausal women. Obesity. 2007 Jan; 15(1):100–6.

[16] Monastyrsky, K. Fiber Menace: The Truth about the Leading Role of Fiber in Diet Failure, Constipation, Hemorrhoids, Irritable Bowel Syndrome, Ulcerative Colitis, Crohn's Disease, and Colon Cancer. Ageless Press, 2005.

[17] Park, Y., et al. High fiber intake linked to reduced breast cancer risk. Am J Clin Nutr. 2009; 90:664–71.

[18] Mozaffarian, D., et al. Effects on coronary heart disease of increasing polyunsaturated fat in place of saturated fat: A systematic review and meta-analysis of randomized controlled trials. PLOSmedicine.org 2010.

[19] Micha, R., Mozaffarian, D. Saturated fat and cardiometabolic risk factors, coronary heart disease, stroke, and diabetes: A fresh look at the evidence. Lipids. 2010 Oct; 45(10):893–905.

[20] Siri-Tarino, P. W., et al. Meta-analysis of prospective cohort studies evaluating the association of saturated fat with cardiovascular disease. Am J Clin Nutr 2010; 91:535–46.

[21] Ramsden, C., et al. Use of dietary linoleic acid for secondary prevention of coronary heart disease and death. BMJ 2013; 346:e8707.

[22] Mayeaux, M., et al. Effects of cooking conditions on the lycopene content in tomatoes. Journal of Food Science. 2006 Sep 9; 71(8):461–64.

[23] Subramanian, S. Fact or fiction: Raw veggies are healthier than cooked ones: Do vegetables lose their nutritional value when heated? Scientific American, 2009 Mar 31; http://www.scientificamerican.com/article.cfm?id=raw-veggies-are-healthier.

Step Five: Add The Blood Code Fitness Principles

[1] http://www.nih.gov/news/pr/aug2001/niddk-08.htm from the Diabetes Prevention Program: US National Institute of Health.

[2] Boulé, N. G., et al. Metformin and Exercise in Type 2 Diabetes: Examining treatment modality interactions. Diabetes Care. 2011 July; 34(7):1469–74.

[3] Orchard T, et al. The effect of metformin and intensive lifestyle intervention on the metabolic syndrome: the Diabetes Prevention Program randomized trial. Ann Intern Med. 2005 Apr 19; 142(8):611–9.

[4] Ciloglu, F., et al. Exercise intensity and its effects on thyroid hormones. Neuroendocrinology Letters 2005 Dec; 26(6):830–4.

[5] Bartke, A. Insulin and aging. Cell Cycle, 2008 Nov 1; 7 (21):3338–43.

[6] Masternak, M. M., et al. Insulin sensitivity as a key mediator of growth hormone actions on longevity. Journals of Gerontology Ser A: Biological Sciences and Medical Sciences, 2009 May; 64(5):516–21.

[7] Rozing, M. P., et al. Human insulin/IGF-1 and familial longevity at middle age. Aging. 2009 Jul 24; 1(8):714–22.

[8] Wijsman, C. A., et al. Familial longevity is marked by enhanced insulin sensitivity. Aging Cell, 2011 Feb; 10(1):114–21.

⁹ Tjønna, A. E. Aerobic interval training vs. continuous moderate exercise as a treatment for the metabolic syndrome: A pilot study. Circulation. 2008 July 22; 118(4):346–54.

¹⁰ Black, L. E., et al. Effects of intensity and volume on insulin sensitivity during acute bouts of resistance training. Journal of Strength and Conditioning Research, 2010; 24(4):1109–16.

¹¹ Dimkpa, U. Post-exercise heart rate recovery: An index of cardiovascular fitness. JEPonline 2009; 12(1):19–22.

¹² Brunner, E. J., et al. Adrenocortical, autonomic, and inflammatory causes of the metabolic syndrome: Nested case-control study. Circulation 106, no. 21 (2002): doi:10.1161/01.CIR.0000038364.26310.BD.

¹³ Jolly, M., et al. Impact of exercise on heart rate recovery. Circulation. 2011 Oct 4; 124(14):1520–6.

¹⁴ Bhammar, D. M., et al. Effects of fractionized and continuous exercise on 24-h ambulatory blood pressure. Med Sci Sports Exerc. 2012 Dec; 44(12):2270–6.

¹⁵ Crane, P., et al. Glucose levels and risk of dementia. N Engl J Med. 2013;369:540-548.

¹⁶ Duck-chul, L., et al. Changes in fitness and fatness on the development of cardiovascular disease risk factors: hypertension, metabolic syndrome, and hypercholesterolemia. Journal of the American College of Cardiology. 2012 Feb 14; 665–72.

¹⁷ Kay, A. D., Blazevich, A. J. Effect of acute static stretch on maximal muscle performance: A systematic review. Med Sci Sports Exerc. 2012 Jan; 44(1):154–64.

¹⁸ Morton, S. K., et al. Resistance training vs. static stretching: Effects on flexibility and strength. J Strength Cond Res. 2011 Dec; 25(12):3391–8.

Step Six: Ensure Nutritional Support

¹ Volpe, S. L. Magnesium, the metabolic syndrome, insulin resistance, and type 2 diabetes mellitus. Crit Rev Food Sci Nutr. 2008; 48:293–300.

[1] Farvid, M. S., et al. Comparison of the effects of vitamins and/or mineral supplementation on glomerular and tubular dysfunction in type 2 diabetes. Diabetes Care. 2005 Oct 28; (10):2458–64.

[3] Farvid, M. S., et al. The impact of vitamins and/or mineral supplementation on blood pressure in type 2 diabetes. J Am Coll Nutr. 2004 Jun; 23(3):272–9.

[4] Farvid, M. S., et al. The impact of vitamin and/or mineral supplementation on lipid profiles in type 2 diabetes. Diabetes Res Clin Pract. 2004 Jul; 65(1):21–8.

[5] Khan, H., et al. Vitamin D, type 2 diabetes and other metabolic outcomes: A systematic review and meta-analysis of prospective studies. Proc Nutr Soc. 2013 Feb; 72(1):89–97.

[6] Alaimo, K., et al. Dietary intake of vitamins, minerals, and fiber of person ages 2 months and over in the United States: Third National Health and Nutrition Examination Survey, Phase 1, 1988–91, Adv Data. 1994; (258):1–28.

[7] National Institutes of Health Office of Dietary Supplements. Magnesium: http://ods.od.nih.gov/factsheets/magnesium.asp. As of January 2013.

[8] Rosolova, H., Mayer, O., Reaven, G. M. Insulin-mediated glucose disposal is decreased in normal subjects with relatively low plasma magnesium concentrations. Metabolism. 2000; 49:418–20.

[9] Paolisso, G., et al. Daily magnesium supplements improve glucose handling in elderly subjects. Am J Clin Nutr. 1992; 55:1161–67.

[10] Slutsky, I., et al. Enhancement of synaptic plasticity through chronically reduced Ca++ flux during uncorrelated activity. Neuron, 2004; 44:835–49.

[11] Evangelopoulos, A. A., et al. An inverse relationship between cumulating components of the metabolic syndrome and serum magnesium levels. Nutrition Res. 2008; 28:659–63.

[12] Xiao, Q., et al. Dietary and supplemental calcium intake and cardiovascular disease mortality. JAMA Intern Med, 2013 Apr 22; 173(8):639–46.

[13] Masharani, U., et al. Chromium supplementation in non-obese non-diabetic subjects is associated with a decline in insulin sensitivity. BMC Endocr Disord. 2012 Nov 30; 12:31.

[14] Balk, E. M., et al. Effect of chromium supplementation on glucose metabolism and lipids: A systematic review of randomized controlled trials. Diabetes Care. 2007 Aug; 30(8):2154–63.

[15] Barklay, L. Low chromium linked to heart disease risk in patients with diabetes. Diabetes Care. 2004; 27:2211–16.

[16] Brøndum-Jacobsen, P., et al. 25-Hydroxyvitamin D and symptomatic ischemic stroke: An original study and meta-analysis. Ann Neurol. 2013 Jan; 73(1):38–47.

[17] Arnson, Y., et al. Vitamin D inflammatory cytokines and coronary events: A comprehensive review. lin Rev Allergy Immunol. 2013 Jan doi: 10.1007/s12016-013-8356-0.

[18] Tsur, A., et al. Decreased serum concentrations of 25-Hydroxycholecalciferol are associated with increased risk of progression to impaired fasting glucose and diabetes. Diabetes Care. 2013 Feb doi; 10.2337/dc12-1050.

[19] George, P. S., et al. Effect of vitamin D supplementation on glycemic control and insulin resistance: a systematic review and meta-analysis. Diabet Med. 2012 Aug; 29(8):e142–50.

[20] Geleijnse, J. M., et al. Dietary intake of menaquinone is associated with a reduced risk of coronary heart disease: the Rotterdam Study. J Nutr. 2004 Nov; 134(11):3100–5.

[21] Yoshida, M., et al. Effect of vitamin K supplementation on insulin resistance in older men and women. Diabetes Care. 2008 Nov; 31(11): 2092–96.

[22] Abeywardena, M., Patten, G. Role of ω3 long-chain polyunsaturated fatty acids in reducing cardio-metabolic risk factors. Endocr Metab Immune Disord Drug Targets. 2011 Sep 1; 11(3):232–46.

[23] Lin, N., et al. Prolonged high iodine intake is associated with inhibition of type 2 deiodinase activity in pituitary and elevation of serum thyrotropin levels. Br J Nutr 2012 Mar; 107(5):674–82.

[24] Gärtner, R., et al. Selenium supplementation in patients with auto-immune thyroiditis decreases thyroid peroxidase antibodies concentrations. J Clin Endocrinol Metab. 2002 Apr; 87(4):1687–91.

[25] Hodgson, J. M., et al. Coenzyme Q10 improves blood pressure and glycemic control: A controlled trial in subjects with type 2 diabetes. Eur J Clin Nutr. 2002 Nov; 56(11):1137–42.

[26] Mezawa, M., et al. The reduced form of coenzyme Q10 improves glycemic control in patients with type 2 diabetes: An open label pilot study. Biofactors. 2012 Nov/Dec; 38(6):416–21.

[27] Tiziani, A. Havard's Nursing Guide to Drugs, 2013.

[28] Dietmar, A., et al. Ubiquinol supplementation enhances peak power production in trained athletes: A double-blind, placebo controlled study. Journal of the International Society of Sports Nutrition 2013, 10:24.

[29] Weber, C., et al. Coenzyme Q10 in the diet—daily intake and relative bioavailability. Mol Aspects Mes. 1997; 18 Suppl:S251–4.

[30] Ansar, H., et al. Effect of alpha-lipoic acid on blood glucose, insulin resistance and glutathione peroxidase of type 2 diabetic patients. Saudi Med J. 2011 Jun; 32(6):584–8.

[31] Kamenova, P. Improvement of insulin sensitivity in patients with type 2 diabetes mellitus after oral administration of alpha-lipoic acid. Hormones (Athens). 2006 Oct/Dec; 5(4):251–8.

[32] Henriksen, E. J. Exercise training and the antioxidant alpha-lipoic acid in the treatment of insulin resistance and type 2 diabetes. Free Radic Biol Med. 2006 Jan 1; 40(1):3–12.

[33] Ibrahimpasic, K. Alpha-lipoic acid and glycaemic control in diabetic neuropathies at type 2 diabetes treatment. Med Arh. 2013; 67(1):7–9.

[34] Zhang, H., Wei, J., Xue, R., et al. Berberine lowers blood glucose in type 2 diabetes mellitus patients through increasing insulin receptor expression. Metabolism 2010; 59:285–92.

[35] Pan, G. Y., et al. Inhibitory action of berberine on glucose absorption. 2003 Dec; 38(12):911–4.

[36] Jun, Y., et al. Efficacy of berberine in patients with type 2 diabetes. Metabolism. 2008 May; 57(5): 712–17.

37 Li, Z. Q., et al. Berberine acutely inhibits the digestion of maltose in the intestine. J Ethnopharmacol. 2012 Jul 13; 142(2):474–80.

38 Baker, W. L., et al. Effect of cinnamon on glucose control and lipid parameters. Diabetes Care. 2008 Jan; 31(1):41–3.

39 Baskaran, K., et al. Antidiabetic effect of a leaf extract from Gymnema sylvestre in non-insulin-dependent diabetes mellitus patients. J Ethnopharmacol 1990; 30:295–305.

40 Vuksan, V., et al. American ginseng (Panax quinquefolius) reduces postprandial glycemia in nondiabetic subjects and subjects with type 2 diabetes mellitus. Arch Intern Med. 2000 Apr 10; 160(7):1009–13.

41 Park, E. Y., et al. Increase in insulin secretion induced by Panax ginseng berry extracts contributes to the amelioration of hyperglycemia in streptozotocin induced diabetic mice. J Ginseng Res. 2012 Apr; 36(2):153–60.

Lifestyle Habits that Support Your Steps: Alcohol, Sleep, and Stress

1 Van Cauter, E., et al. Impact of sleep and sleep loss on neuroendocrine and metabolic function. Horm Res. 2007; 67 Suppl 1:2–9.

2 Nedeltcheva, M. D., Arlet, V. Insufficient sleep undermines dietary efforts to reduce adiposity. Annals of Int Med, vol. 153, no. 7, 2010 Oct 5; 435–41.

3 Spruyt, K., et.al. Sleep duration, sleep regularity, body weight, and metabolic homeostasis in school-aged children, Pediatrics, 2011 Feb; 127(2):e345–52.

4 Kuo, L., et al. Chronic stress, combined with a high-fat/high-sugar diet, shifts sympathetic signaling toward neuropeptide Y and leads to obesity and the metabolic syndrome, Ann N Y Acad Sci. 2008 Dec; 1148:232–37.

5 Raikkonen, K., Matthews, K. A., Kuller, L. H. The relationship between psychological risk attributes and the metabolic syndrome in healthy women: Antecedent or consequence? Metabolism. 2002; 51:1573–77.

Digging Deeper: Confidence through Research

[1] Greene, P., Willett, W., Devecis, J., et al., Pilot 12-week feeding weight-loss comparison: Low-fat vs. low-carbohydrate (ketogenic) diets, abstract presented at the North American Association for the Study of Obesity Annual Meeting 2003, Obesity Research.

[2] Shai, I., Schwarzfuchs, D., Henkin, Y., et al. Weight loss with a low-carbohydrate, Mediterranean, or low-fat diet. N Engl J Med. 2008; 359:229–41.

[3] Estruch, R., et al. Primary prevention of cardiovascular disease with a Mediterranean diet. N Engl J Med. 2013 Apr 4; 368(14):1279–90.

[4] Ajala, O., et al. Systematic review and meta-analysis of different dietary approaches to the management of type 2 diabetes. Am J Clin Nutr. 2013 Mar; 97(3):505–16.

[5] Shai, I., et al. Dietary intervention to reverse carotid atherosclerosis. Circulation. 2010 Mar 16; 121(10):1200–8.

[6] Shai, I., et al. Weight Loss with a Low-Carbohydrate, Mediterranean, or Low-Fat Diet. N Engl J Med 2008; 359:229–41.

[7] Nystrom, F. Publication database is found at: http://www.imh.liu.se/kardiovaskular-medicin/staff/fredrik-nystrom?l=en

[8] Sinatra, S., Bowden, J. The Great Cholesterol Myth: Why Lowering Your Cholesterol Won't Prevent Heart Disease-and the Statin-Free Plan That Will, Fair Winds Press, 2012.

[9] Forman, J., et al. Uric acid and insulin sensitivity and risk of incident hypertension. Arch Intern Med. 2009; 169(2):155–62.

[10] Jackson, P., et al. Statins for primary prevention: At what coronary risk is safety assured? British Journal of Clinical Pharmacology, 2001 52:439–46.

[11] Abramson, J., Wright, J. Are lipid-lowering guidelines evidence-based? Lancet, vol. 369, 2007 Jan 20; 369(9557):168–9.

[12] Reaven, M. D., Gerald, T. K., Fox, B. Syndrome X: The Silent Killer; The New Heart Disease Risk. Simon & Schuster, 2001.

[13]   Jeppesen, J., et al. Low triglycerides-high high-density lipoprotein cholesterol and risk of ischemic heart disease. Arch Intern Med. 2001; 161:361–66.

[14]   Lakka, H., et al. Hyperinsulinemia and the risk of cardiovascular death and acute coronary and cerebrovascular events in men. Arch Intern Med. 2000; 160(8):1160–68.

[15]   Gunter, M., et al. Insulin, insulin-like growth factor-I, and risk of breast cancer in postmenopausal women. Natl Cancer Inst. 2009 Jan 7; 101(1):48–60.

[16]   Antoniadis, A. G., et al. Insulin resistance in relation to melanoma risk. Melanoma Res., vol. 21(6). 2011 Dec; 541–46.

[17]   Giovannucci, E. Metabolic syndrome, hyperinsulinemia, and colon cancer: A review. Am J Clin Nutr, vol. 86, no. 3, 2007 Sept; 836–42.

[18]   Rocchin, A. P., et al. Insulin and renal sodium retention in obese adolescents. Hypertension. 1989; 14:367–74.

[19]   Festa, A., et al. LDL particle size in relation to insulin, proinsulin, and insulin sensitivity. The Insulin Resistance Atherosclerosis Study. Diabetes Care. 1999 Oct; 22(10):1688–93.

[20]   Targher, G., et al. Risk of cardiovascular disease in patients with non-alcoholic fatty liver disease. N Engl J Med. 2010 Sep 30; 363(14):1341–50.

[21]   Tock, L. Nonalcoholic fatty liver disease decrease in obese adolescents after multidisciplinary therapy, European Journal of Gastroenterology and Hepatology, vol. 18, no. 12, 2006; 1241–45.

[22]   Machado, M., Non-alcoholic fatty liver disease and insulin resistance, European Journal of Gastroenterology and Hepatology, vol. 17, no. 8, 2005; 823–26.

[23]   Masternak, M., et al. Insulin sensitivity as a key mediator of growth hormone actions on longevity. J Gerontol A Biol Sci Med Sci. 2009 May; 64A(5): 516–21.

[24]   http://www.nhlbi.nih.gov/news/press-releases/2008/accord-clinical-trial-publishes-results.html: The Accord Trial report from the US National Institutes of Health, 2008.

[25] Guyton and Hall. Textbook of Medical Physiology, 12th edition. Saunders, 2010.

[26] Oh, J. Y. Regional adiposity, adipokines, and insulin resistance in type 2 diabetes. Metab J. 2012 Dec; 36(6):412–14.

[27] Renaldi, O., et al. Hypoadiponectinemia: a risk factor for metabolic syndrome. Acta Med Indones. 2009 Jan; 41(1):20–4.

[28] Sapolsky, R. Why Zebras Don't Get Ulcers, 3rd edition. Holt Paperbacks, 2004.

Staying in Your Sweet Spot

[1] Ryan, A. Insulin resistance with aging: Effects of diet and exercise. Sports Med. 2000 Nov; 30(5):327–46.

Index

free triiodothyronine (Free T3, FT3).
See triiodothyronine, free
frequency of meals, 151, 156
fructose (simple sugar), 109–112,
232, 234
fruits, 102, 109, 111, 115

G

galactose (simple sugar), 110
gestational diabetes, 39
glipizide (Glucotrol), 210, 232
glossary, 230–235
glucagon, 213, 215, 232, 233
Glucophage. See metformin
glucose (simple sugar), 110
Glucotrol (glipizide), 210, 232
gluten grains, 122
glycemic index, 109–110, 232
glycosylated hemoglobin. See
HgbA1C
goiter, 232
goitrogens, 96, 232; see also
cruciferous vegetables
gout, 76, 209
grains/breads, 120–123, 218–223
gluten, 120–122
non-gluten, 120–121
to avoid, 122–123
whole-grain foods, 120–121,
153
granola, 122, 218

H

Hashimoto's thyroiditis, 52, 232
HDL. See high-density lipoprotein
health-care providers
and blood pressure medications,
228
and blood tests, 19, 24, 27,
30–52, 208
and fitness, 170
and nutritional support, 177,
183, 193
and thyroid prescriptions, 94, 99
heart disease
and alcohol, 197
and body fat, 56, 64, 90
and diet, 129, 143, 154–157, 182,
185, 204, 206
and exercise, 166, 172
links to risk of, 31, 37, 45, 47, 56,
71, 93
risk assessment, 41
and stress, 200
hematocrit (HCT), 32
hemoglobin (HGB), 32
Hemoglobin A1C. See HgbA1C
Hemogram. See Complete Blood
Count
herbal therapies, 190–193
American ginseng, 191–192
berberine extract, 190–191
and blood sugar metabolism,
190–193

"inflammation" test (hs-CRP). *See*
C-Reactive Protein
insoluble fiber, 113–114, 120,
152–153
insulin, high. *See* high insulin
insulin, low. *See* low insulin
insulin resistance (IR), 73–92,
233
and action steps ahead of you,
82–84
an advantage, 80–81
and body fat, 71–72
case study: IR / metabolic
syndrome, 85–86
clinical conditions, 76
and fitness, 159–160
and high insulin/hypothyroid,
73–100
nondiabetic conditions, 76
treating glucose and not IR,
209–211
what it means for you, 79–81
insulin sensitivity, 209, 233
and blood tests, 38
and body fat, 57
and fitness principles, 50, 159,
163, 166
and nutrients, 181, 184–185, 189
and transition to insulin
resistance, 89
interval training, 75, 83, 163, 165–168,
170–171
iodine, 48–49, 96–97, 176, 186, 232

K

kale, 96, 115, 117, 177, 184, 220–221,
224, 226
kidney function, 36, 179, 209
kidney stones, 115

L

LADA (diabetes type 1.5), 38
large meal size, 124–125
leafy greens, dark, 115, 155, 181,
184–185, 218, 224
legumes/beans, 114, 118–120, 153,
181, 234
leptin, 211–213, 230, 233
leptin resistance, 212
leukocytes. *See* white blood cells
Lifestyle Habits that Support Your
Steps, 194–202
alcohol, 194–197;
see also alcohol
sleep, 198–199
stress, 200–202
linoleic acid, 155
lipid panels, 26,40–42, 179, 199
liver disease, fatty, 26, 35, 76, 195,
209, 231
liver enzymes, 26, 35, 89, 231
low blood glucose. *See*
hypoglycemia
low blood sugar. *See* hypoglycemia

15146688R00167

Made in the USA
Middletown, DE
25 October 2014